THE EFFORTLESS SLEEP METHOD

Effortless Sleep Products
sasha@effortless-sleep.com

First Edition

The author and publisher of this material make no medical claims for its use. This material is not intended to treat, diagnose nor cure any illness. If you need medical attention, please consult your doctor.

THE EFFORTLESS SLEEP METHOD

The Incredible New Cure for Insomnia and Chronic Sleep Problems

Sasha Stephens

CONTENTS

PREFACE

Part One –
GROUNDWORK

Part Two –
THE MEDICAL PROFESSION AND STANDARD
APPROACHES TO TREATING INSOMNIA

Part Three -
PRELIMINARIES AND PHILOSOPHY

Part Four -
THE MAKING OF A MONSTER

Part Five -
THE CURE

PREFACE

By Sasha Stephens, Bsc, MA,
Creator of the Effortless Sleep Method™, Sleep Therapist,
Recovered insomniac

I understand

There is no need for you to tell me how bad your insomnia problem is.

I know

I know what you are going through. I *really* know what you are going through. I have experienced the full horror of chronic, long-term insomnia.

I know

I know the way that insomnia feels like a curse, a disease, an affliction which infects every part of your life. I know that it can take over your life, ruin your life, and ultimately *be* your life. I know the desperate, panicky, desolate, pitiful loneliness of lying awake at night and the living hell of going through day after day of work and social activities having not slept. I have wept, prayed, begged, raged, broken down, given up, and been left numb by insomnia.

I know

I have tried the herbs, the Valerian, the Passiflora, the 5HTP, the melatonin, the positive thinking, the wishful thinking, the antihistamines, the vitamin B complex, the zinc supplements, the turkey sandwiches, the exercise before breakfast, the exercise six hours before bed, the relaxation cds, the hypnosis, the sleeping pills, the sleep restriction, the milky drinks, the lavender pillows, the magnetic coils under my mattress, the crystals, the fan in the room, the ioniser in the room, the earplugs, the eye shades, and I've lost count of how many wild and wacky therapies and therapists. *So* many therapists!

I know

I have made silent pleas to God, offered up deals to the universe to exchange everything I own for the ability to sleep. I would have taken heroin if I thought it would make me sleep. I would have sold my soul to the devil if he had asked.

I know

In the deafening, screaming blackness of the sleepless night, I discovered that the fundamental state of the insomniac is one of profound *loneliness*. By night, insomnia separates you from the gently slumbering world of normal sleepers. By day it isolates you from the bustling world of active, happy people. Locked in a bubble of misery, the day of the sleep-deprived person is a semi-real nightmare – a half-life, a non-life.

As insomniacs we have two choices when it comes to normal, everyday work and social activities: we either complain to a largely non-understanding and sometimes unsympathetic social circle, *I didn't sleep well, I can't stay long, I don't think I'm up to that, sorry I'm not on top form today.* Or we learn to 'fake it' – to smile through the misery, to hide the secret truth *I feel like death, I don't want to be here, if you knew how tired I feel, why can't I feel like you do, why can't I enjoy life? What's wrong with me?*

Insomnia may seem almost to have a life of its own, an autonomous persona, or a self-sabotaging part of you over which you have no control; a monster, a possessing demon which taunts you by day and tortures you by night. This cruel tormentor judges you unworthy, undeserving of sleep and punishes you, over and over and over, night after night after night. A sadist, a bully: insomnia is ruthless...and relentless.

I feel your pain like no doctor or therapist, or well-meaning family member has ever done, I feel your pain like only a fellow insomniac can. Because I know how you have suffered, and how you still suffer, I want nothing more than to help you. It breaks my heart to hear about the appalling advice given to insomniacs, and the insensitive and downright negligent way in which they are sometimes treated by the medical profession; treatments which bring with them a whole plethora of new problems and which, unbelievably, often *make the sleeping worse*.

But now, my friend, *it stops here!* Your battle with insomnia is over. I am about to give you your life back. It is time to share with you, the gold – the treasure which took a decade and a half to discover. Using exactly the methods laid out in this book I kicked a *15 year* chronic insomnia problem and now sleep better than I did even as a child. Follow this programme, and you can turn your back on insomnia for good.

I will not disappoint ...

...1...

GROUNDWORK

CHAPTER ONE

My Story

Introduction

Over the years, my experience has led me to believe that it is only those who have suffered themselves who can really understand the particular psychology of chronic insomnia. So before I start teaching you how to get your life back, I want to spend a little while talking about the history of my sleeping problem. Reading about the experience of a fellow sufferer will assure you that what you feel, I have felt, what you suffer, I have suffered. But I do not do this in order that we can commiserate with each other; I do this so that you will believe that no matter how bad your problem is, *you can get better.* So, while you read my story of woe, hold this exciting thought in mind: *this person is now sleeping perfectly, effortlessly, every night!*

How It All Began

For twenty three years I had never really thought about sleep. Although even as a child I always took a fair while (up to an hour) to fall asleep, this fact had never really bothered me. Sleeping was something which happened every night, something I didn't question or wonder about, a part of my life like breathing or walking. Even in a strange bed, on a floor or in a tent, it might take some time, but eventually, I would always drop off.

Things only began to change when I went to university at the age of 23. This was a time of late-night parties and numerous 'free days', all of which meant that for the first time since starting school (when I had regularly got up at 6.30am) I had no set waking-up time. Years later I would find out that for many insomniacs, the problems begin at a time in life when they are keeping irregular hours. For example, during periods of self-employment, unemployment, or when at university. To make matters worse, on those 'free days' where I had no lectures, like the stereotypical student, I would often lie in until noon, 1pm or longer. This meant that on many days I was spending far too long in bed and in a sense, I was getting far *too much* sleep.

A second factor in the development of my insomnia came from my social life which at this time was a whirl of parties and fun events. In order to get a good night's sleep in preparation for one of these social engagements, the day before I would go to bed nice and early at 10.30 or 11pm. The problem was that I might have lain in bed 'til noon that day, so was going to bed only nine hours after getting up! Not being remotely sleepy when I went to bed, combined with anticipation and excitement about the next day meant that I was taking hours and hours to fall asleep.

A Pattern Sets In

Soon I started to notice a pattern of not sleeping well before parties. This was worrying – feeling tired and tense was affecting my ability to enjoy myself. Before long, the same thing started happening before other fun events – weddings, Christmas, picnics, and days out in the country. Irritation soon turned to worry and I started not to be able to look forward to these events quite as much as I once had.

Then one night the whole thing took a turn for the worse. I remember lying in bed on one not particularly special or significant night when the thought flashed through my mind – 'Wouldn't it be awful if I couldn't sleep well tonight, just like on those "special" nights? In fact, what if I didn't sleep at all tonight?' This distressing idea actually began to wake me up. This idea turned to fear, and the further away sleep became. At that moment I noticed for the first time that worrying about not sleeping could keep me awake! And with that, my life changed forever. That night was my first full sleepless night and the beginning of my first long bout of insomnia ...

The next day I had my first experience of the 'morning after'. Little did I know that this was merely a taster of what my life was to become. I lay in bed until 11am before getting up, exhausted and grumpy. All day I could think of nothing but getting some sleep and tried, unsuccessfully, to have a nap in the afternoon. Finally, the evening came and I went to bed early to catch up on all that lost sleep. This time I tried *really* hard to fall asleep ... and I spent another night awake ... and then another, and another! Now I really began to panic. Previously, I had never missed a night's sleep in my life! What was wrong with me? I reasoned that there was only thing I could do: I would go to bed as early as possible and just *stay* there. If I lay there for long enough, I would have to fall asleep, wouldn't I? I decided to simply lie in bed 'until I slept' – for days if necessary!

Oh my goodness! How wrong I was! The longer I lay there, the more tense I became. I ended up with stiff joints and an aching neck and shoulders through unconsciously holding my body still and tense. For weeks I kept up this terrible pattern – lying in bed for as long as possible and trying as hard as I could to fall asleep. Let me just say at this point: if you currently have any notion that the key to sleeping better is to stay in bed longer then I cannot say forcefully enough just how *wrong* this reasoning is! Sometimes I would manage to get an hour's nap on the sofa in the afternoon, or fall asleep in the library with a book on my head. These naps were the only times when I got really sound sleep and they seemed to be enough to sustain me ... just. But night time had become nothing more than one long, angry doze with a pounding heart and a frown on my face.

'Go and See Your Doctor'

I was desperate. I needed help and it was at this point that I made my first big mistake. I did what everyone advises us to do. I did what we are supposed to do. I went to see my doctor.

Knowing what I know today, I still sometimes feel a little bitter about the advice given on that fateful day. Sadly, I know that the same terrible advice given to me all those years ago is still being dished out every day to hundreds of 'fledgling insomniacs'. I now know that at such an early stage, with a few simple modifications to my behaviour I could have broken that silly pattern, stopping this problem in its tracks, and 15 years of suffering could have been avoided. Do you think simple behaviour modification is what my doctor recommended? No, of course it wasn't. She did what doctors do best – she gave me pills.

I was excited at the thought of my first ever sleeping pill – temazepam, also known as Restoril, one of the benzodiazepine family of drugs. It seemed fun, a bit risqué, a legal 'drug' with the power to send you to sleep. I also believed that all my problems were over, that I'd wake up tomorrow, feeling great with all this sorry business behind me. That night I took my first ever temazepam and fell asleep quickly, or rather, I fell unconscious quickly. I was surprised to awaken in the morning quite early, not refreshed and energetic, but with a feeling of thick-headed grogginess – my first ever sleeping pill hangover. As the day went on, I expected to perk up a bit but this never happened. The groggy feeling lasted all day and was almost enough to put me off taking another pill. However, the next night the same thing happened. I got up in the morning feeling no better than when I had missed a night's sleep and it was difficult to work out whether I preferred the feeling of sleep deprivation or the hangover from the temazepam. I took temazepam for only a couple more days before it stopped working; it was no longer succeeding in sending me to sleep, and the night long 'angry dozing' was back. I then discovered that there is a feeling *worse* than either sleep deprivation or sleeping pill hangover: the combination of the two! In 15 years, I have never read a book, an article or heard any mention from any medical professional, or in any medical journal, of the horror of this experience. As you may well know, the feeling of sleep deprivation *combined* with a sleeping pill hangover is horrific, desperate, and worse than anything that insomnia alone can make a person feel.

I went back to my doctor to tell her about my surprising lack of success with temazepam. Unbelievably, nitrazepam was quickly to follow. Nitrazepam, also known as Mogadon, is almost never prescribed for insomnia in the UK any more as it is highly addictive, but this was 1993 and there were still unscrupulous doctors willing to offer it. Unlike temazepam, nitrazepam knocked me out like a sledgehammer. There was no dozing here, I was unconscious. The next day the hangover was still present but was not as bad, better than with temazepam. I took the nitrazepam for about a fortnight after which the same thing happened as had done with temazepam. I found that I could stay awake all night and was only managing to fall into a light doze. I needed a higher dose, which I took, and which worked.

I had had to increase my dose after a fortnight! I realised immediately that this drug had the potential to be horribly addictive and stopped taking it. *I was one of the lucky ones.* If I had not had the presence of mind and the good fortune to stop taking the nitrazepam of my own accord, I might have had a very different story to tell – and it might not have been a recovery story!

On the third visit to the doctor I refused any more sleeping pills and a different approach was taken. This was the time of the birth of a new wonder drug – a panacea which had the capability of curing depression for ever with no side-effects. So effective was this drug that many intelligent people actually spoke of putting it in the water supply in order to make the world a happier place.

Prozac – 'The Wonder Drug'

"Insomnia is a sign of depression," the doctor told me. "Take Prozac and your sleep will improve." I had never complained of depression. I was feeling worried about the lack of sleep, but I still considered myself to be a reasonably happy person. However, I trusted the doctor and went home with my Prozac. Being an anti-depressant, Prozac would take at least two weeks to start working and I took it for several months before I realised the effect it was starting to have. It induced what can only be described as a gradually increasing paranoia and sense of dread, an underlying feeling that 'something was always very wrong', which I had never before experienced. It is not an exaggeration to say that my general mental state and my sleeping actually deteriorated! Prozac is supposed to make you feel happier by balancing serotonin levels which are often depleted in depressed people. But the sad truth is that for many people (perhaps those who never had a serotonin imbalance in the first place) it can have a very negative effect.

On my next visit, I saw a different doctor, a man this time. He took a very different approach which did not involve sending me away with a new bottle of pills. He took my problem very seriously and referred me to a psychiatrist. But there would be a long wait … After six months of appalling sleep, I finally got my psychiatrist's appointment.

A Psychiatrist's Advice

This psychiatrist knew as much about sleep problems as I did about particle physics, perhaps less. After a very thorough and intrusive investigation into my past, my childhood, my relationship with my parents, siblings and partners, my every thought, he concluded by saying 'I can offer you two things – drug treatment or psychoanalysis, and I don't think either is going to help you.' I was devastated. It was as if I had tried all that the medical profession had to offer and nothing could help. It was at this point that I started to form an inconceivably destructive belief, one that would be with me for many years: I was incurable, my problem was no like other person's. I was different.

And so my insomnia remained and life went on, if you could call it living …

The Online Information Explosion

Then in 1996 something monumental happened which was to dominate and control my sleeping patterns and behaviour for the next ten years. I got access to the internet for the first time and the whole world with all its sleep cures was now at my fingertips.

I started looking into alternative sleep treatments, pouring money into all manner of sleep cures, including hypnosis, meditation, acupuncture and a myriad of herbs, pills and potions. But nothing ever seemed to make any difference. Every remedy I tried was supposed to improve sleep, but not mine, it seemed. It was as if my body was automatically rejecting anything that was supposed to help me sleep. Any herb or pill I would fight, any relaxation technique would wake me up. It was at this point that I first tried Sleep Restriction Therapy. Tragically, this experience was so disastrous that it put me off *all* behaviour modification for over a decade. And so my bad sleeping habits continued unchecked.

As I tested each new thing and rejected it, one belief kept on growing

My problem is different.

Is this starting to sound familiar..?

Finding the Online Insomnia Community

Not only did I discover that there were literally thousands of new cures and remedies to try, I also discovered a worldwide community of insomniacs like myself. How wonderful to find a whole new community of sympathetic, empathetic, well-meaning friends who could understand exactly what I was going through. We would write to each other by email and on forum sites. We would converse and commiserate, tell our tales, suggest remedies and offer sympathy when they didn't work. I was no longer alone! There were insomniacs like me all over the world, millions of them, all suffering just like me, just like *you!*

I even started to hear from people whose problems were worse than mine! Some people were desperately addicted to sleeping pills, some people apparently didn't sleep at all, and most amazingly – some people had suffered for 30 years! While listening to all these tales of woe a strange thing started to happen... rather than be encouraged by the few success stories, or comforted that in comparison my problem was not so bad, I instead found myself completely identifying with these people and their terrible situations. Perhaps this has happened to you, too. Their stories terrified me! All I could think was that my future had exactly the same in store. Their fears soon became *my* fears, and before long, their problems became mine too.

My life had now altered beyond all recognition. My obsession had grown to unhealthy levels and every moment of my life was now ruled by thoughts about sleep. From the time I got up, what I ate, what I drank, whether and when I exercised, whether and when I drank coffee, or cola, all these simple decisions could not be made without taking into account their possible effect on my sleep.

And then there were daily dilemmas about sleep remedies - should I take a Nytol, should I not, should I meditate before bed, what should I read, what should I watch on television, should I get drunk, should I avoid water in case I woke up needing the loo? Should I, should I, should I? Every decision of my life had to pass the self-imposed 'will it affect my sleep?' filter.

Making plans went completely out of the window. I stopped going on holiday. I avoided staying with friends and never invited people to my home. I still had a social life but activities needed to be spontaneous decisions made on the same day. I wouldn't dare suggest meeting a friend for lunch, a weekend picnic or even a shopping trip. Looking back, I am amazed that my friends continued to bother with me at all.

Insomnia had taken over my entire life and I was now set in a pattern which was to last another ten years. On occasion I would get a really good night, tantalising me with the sheer joy of a life without exhaustion. But these were rare – most nights were spent in a light doze, giving me just enough sleep to survive but not enough to ever really feel OK. And, on those 'special nights' when I had something important or exciting to get up for, I would get no sleep at all.

The New Non-benzodiazepines

Despite my disastrous experience with pills, I still couldn't give up the idea that some sort of pill might just work for me. Especially as I now had a new doctor, one who was very free with her prescription-writing pen. She was very enthusiastic about a whole new range of sleeping pills which were completely different to all others that had gone before. These were the so-called non-benzodiazepines, which apparently came without any of the addictive qualities and terrible side-effects of the previous benzodiazepine-based drugs. My doctor prescribed zopiclone, commonly known as Zimovane or Imovane. Again, I was moderately excited about this new drug and took it with some hope. The zopiclone gave me about two hours of thick-headed unconsciousness from which I woke feeling like I hadn't slept at all. But most shocking, once again, was the morning's hangover. I had plunged into an instant waking pit of despair, which lasted most of the day. I only took the drug for two nights. I would never take it again, the effect was too horrible. But my doctor and her busy pen were not finished yet. She had the perfect drug, one that worked quickly but, because it wore off in a few hours, the hangover problem would be eliminated. This drug was the romantically named Sonata (zaleplon). Unfortunately, Sonata was to have almost no effect at all. Sometimes I did manage to fall asleep, but with the added side-effect of waking me very early in the morning, wide awake and unable to get back to sleep. The following day I would still be left groggy and unsatisfied. So much for Sonata the wonder drug.

No More Pills

At this point I made a decision – I would *never* again take a sleeping pill. I can categorically say that in 15 years, no sleeping pill whatsoever has given me a good night's sleep without a hangover. I will go further in saying that in 15 years, there has never been a drug whose effects were preferable to a night without sleep! The rule for me seemed to be *no sleep is better than drugged sleep*.

What is most astonishing is that at this point not one health professional, even the psychiatrist, had ever asked me about my sleeping behaviour. I still had no idea that lying in bed in the morning, for example, far from helping, was actually contributing to the problem.

Sometimes I would decide that I would completely ignore the problem, act like it wasn't there with the thought that eventually, it would go away of its own accord. I would resolve to 'stop letting it take over my life, I would be happy no matter what, I would go on holiday, I would enjoy a camping trip with friends and no bloody insomnia was going to stop me!' And away I would go with my friends, with all good intentions, perhaps to a weekend summer festival. Three miserable days later, having missed three full nights of sleep, I would go home early, tearful and exhausted.

The opposite mood was complete desperation. All I wanted was to be normal. Sometimes I would pray, although I had no religious beliefs. I would cry and rage, scream at myself, scream at God, scream at my partner who had dared to arrange a dinner party at the weekend. I was completely obsessed. I hope you are beginning to get an idea of just how crazy this sleeping problem had made me. At the height of my problem, every part of my life, every decision I ever made was in some way related to sleep, or the lack of it. Insomnia didn't just rule my life. Insomnia was my life …

Turning The Corner

It was in 2005 that things changed for me when a friend convinced me to go on a fortnight's activity holiday in the countryside. The weeks leading up to this trip were ridden with anxiety. What if I didn't sleep at all for two weeks? Would I be able to enjoy myself? I packed every sleep remedy and aid I could think of, pillows, drugs, earplugs, herbs and mp3 player loaded with all number of relaxation recordings …

When I arrived I was in for a shock. The schedule was so strict that there was no time for naps or lie-ins. And, horror of horrors, I had to share a room with three other people. This was intolerable! What if one of them snored? What if they got up and disturbed me in the night? I complained to the organisers about my sleeping arrangements and told them of my problem. I tried to make them understand that my requirements were *different* from those of ordinary people. This was no *ordinary* sleeping problem – I *had* to have a private room! Unimpressed by my hysterical demands, the organisers told me there was no other place to sleep.

I would never have been able to predict what then happened and the totally unexpected effect it would have on my sleep. We all had to get out of bed at 6am, had little free time and were kept awake throughout the day. I didn't sleep for the first couple of nights which was hard. But with so much going on, there was little time to fret about lost sleep. I actually found myself forgetting about my tiredness and started to enjoy myself. In addition to this, because I knew that these 'important' nights were going to continue for some time, I stopped stressing about them. I *had* to get out of bed and get involved in the social events. I couldn't make excuses for not going, I couldn't tell myself 'it'll be over this time tomorrow', like I normally would. I couldn't engage in my normal routines, and no one was going to take any notice of my demands. There was literally nothing I could do. After a few days, I actually started to forget about my sleeping problem. At bedtime I was sleepy and exhausted … and so I began to sleep.

On the way home from this thoroughly enjoyable fortnight, I reflected on my incredible success with sleeping. During this fortnight I had been unable to engage in my normal insomnia-confirming behaviour and also had been forced into externally-imposed 'sleep hygiene' (this will be explained in detail in Part 3). I was prevented from carrying out my usual obsessive routines and had no audience for my tales of sleeplessness. I had always known that my negative thoughts were a hindrance to any recovery, but until now I hadn't realised how connected these thoughts were to my *behaviour* concerning sleep.

Suddenly I saw the problem in a completely new light. In a flash I realised all the things I was doing wrong, all the ways in which *I was enabling my insomnia!* I could see that the combination of poor sleep habits, negative thoughts and associated behaviour was maintaining the problem, holding it firmly in place. *This* is why no insomnia cures or sleep remedies ever worked for me: *I was doing this to myself!* The solution was clear to me and I *knew* I could get over the problem. I hadn't yet found the Holy Grail, but I knew I was on the right road. I had turned a corner with my insomnia and

I was never to look back. In a nutshell, I realised that we *must* take a holistic approach to insomnia. Not treating sleep itself in isolation, as doctors do with sleeping pills, but rather by attending to thoughts and beliefs about sleep, and to habits and behaviours which create and reinforce the problem.

Beginning to Write

I started writing things down, any new insight or observation. And so my knowledge and understanding of insomnia grew. Rapidly, my sleeping improved, often surprising me in circumstances where I once would never have expected to sleep. When my online insomnia email friends around the world heard of my recovery, they began begging me for advice. And so I began sharing it with people as best I could. My nights were now taken up writing motivational emails to my insomniac friends. I had no medical training whatsoever, and yet the advice I was able to offer was gratefully received, even by those who had attended the most elite sleep clinics. I had unwittingly become a sleep therapist! Time and time again, I was begged to write a book about my recovery, putting all my good advice down in one place. And so I did. I began to formulate a set of rules, guidelines and advice which was eventually to become the Effortless Sleep Method.

I now sell a range of sleep-related products, including sleep boosters, sleep inducers and stress relievers. I also run workshops and seminars in which you can deepen your understanding of the Method. Find out more at www.sashastephens.com. Here you can also subscribe to *The Good Sleepers' Club* and receive free daily snippets of sleepy wisdom from my famous *Bedtime Stories*.

Personal consultations by email, Skype and in person are sometimes available. See the website for details.

All of my sleep products are available at greatly reduced prices to readers. Visit www.sashastephens.com/discount to access the special prices. This page is hidden from normal view and the address is made available only to readers of this book.

A Word of Warning ...!

When reading this book, don't skip sections! Careful planning has gone into the ordering of the chapters and the book should be read from start to finish, in the order in which it is written. There are good reasons for this: to start with, the advice is cumulative. Some of the most important messages build on insights from earlier chapters and will make little sense if the earlier sections have not been read. Under no circumstances should you skip to the 'cure' section. You will not get the full benefit of any particular guideline if you have not fully understood why it has been suggested. Without some understanding of the *reasons* for the advice given, *this programme will not work for you.*

You may be the type of person who skips sections, or picks and chooses the advice to follow, perhaps because you have done some research yourself. You may be very 'in touch' with your problem and therefore feel you have a very good idea of what is or isn't likely to work. If this is so, then *you of all people* must follow *all* the advice. One very clear pattern in chronic insomnia is that the 'I know best' attitude contributes massively to the severity of the problem, and hinders any recovery. If your recovery turns out to be like that of most people, you will find yourself being astonished by the unexpected things which turn out to help and the odd twists which lead to new understanding. By skipping sections you run the risk of missing a vital piece of information which could be key in your recovery. What is more, it is likely that *almost everything you think you know about your problem and the best way to treat it will turn out to be false!* Think about it: if you really understood your problem, you wouldn't be reading this book!

Don't let this become yet another 'one that didn't work', simply because you don't follow the instructions properly.

...2...

THE MEDICAL PROFESSION AND STANDARD APPROACHES TO TREATING INSOMNIA

- CHAPTER TWO -

The Medical Profession and Standard Approaches to Treating Insomnia

Introduction

If you are a long-term sufferer you will almost certainly have tried many cures and remedies, both conventional and 'alternative'. In this section I will describe the standard treatments for insomnia by conventional medicine. I will also suggest in this section reasons why these are often unsuccessful. If you are one of those people for whom 'nothing seems to work' then this section will be very important for you. On the other hand, if your insomnia is a recent problem, you may be bewildered by the sheer number of sleeping remedies available and you may be thinking about asking your doctor for a sleeping pill. Be warned, the philosophy behind the Effortless Sleep Method is completely incompatible with the taking of hypnotic sleeping drugs; this section is dedicated to showing you why.

'It Takes One to Know One'

I am convinced that only those who have really suffered can understand the particular psychology of insomnia. One reason for this belief is that many medical explanations and attitudes seem to show little insight into the problem itself, particularly in terms of the consequences of insomnia and the way it can negatively affect a person's life. Consider, for example, the following statement taken from one current, well-known sleep clinic's online programme.

'People worry unnecessarily about the effect that a night without sleep will have on the following day. Tests show that performance is hardly affected by lack of sleep and the worst that can happen is that your mood will be affected.'

This advice is supposed to reassure us that our worst fears for the following day are unfounded. The implication seems to be that insomnia is only a problem insofar as it affects our productivity and efficiency, that mood is unimportant so long as we can still produce the same output. In other words, if the boss is satisfied, a little thing like a bad mood is irrelevant. With so little understanding of the debilitating effects of insomnia, it is statements like this that make me wonder whether their authors have ever known the utter misery of a missed night's sleep. Could anyone who has experienced the waking hell of sleep deprivation suggest that mood is a minor consideration? Mood is not a small thing, mood is *every*thing.

But when it comes to treating the condition, this lack of understanding is even more apparent. The first part of this chapter is devoted to the subject of sleeping pills and you are advised to read it thoroughly. Even if you think you have heard all there is to know on the matter, you may well learn something new. I am not a medical doctor, but in my opinion, nothing reveals the misunderstanding of sleep problems as much as the prescribing of hypnotic sleeping pills for long-term insomnia.

'Can't You Give Me Something to Make Me Sleep?'

Medical knowledge in many areas of human health is truly awe-inspiring and some members of my immediate family certainly would not be alive today without the quick and brilliant actions of doctors. However, the more incredible doctors become at treating severe illness, the greater becomes our expectation that they should be able to cure any problem which may affect our lives. We often imagine that there must be a medical solution, in other words, a *drug* solution, to every problem. The truth is that in the vast majority of cases, insomnia does not have any 'physical' cause. This means that going to a medical doctor with a sleeping problem is a little like going with a broken heart and any drug treatment is hardly likely to be effective!

My feeling is that the medical profession in Britain, Europe, America and the western world in general has not always adequately acknowledged the significance of *belief* in cases of insomnia. Of course the placebo effect is well-recognised by doctors but when it comes to insomnia this goes way beyond the usual 'positive-thinking-aids-recovery' effect. Sleep can be such a fragile and elusive thing that belief can literally make the difference between sleeping and not. When treating insomnia, it is vital to instil a natural trust in *one's own ability to sleep*. It is because of this fact that I now feel that any doctor who prescribes a drug for moderate to long-term insomnia has not fully understood the condition.

My absolute conviction is that the drug paradigm is completely *wrong* for the treatment of insomnia.

CHAPTER THREE

Some Facts about Sleeping Pills

Sleeping Pills and Quality – The Stages of Sleep

A full night of quality sleep is a complicated issue and the terms 'awake' and 'asleep' do not fully capture or do justice to the complexity of the various levels of consciousness that are had in a single night. Sleep actually comes in at least three types, or 'stages', each of which is quite distinct from the others.

Stage 1 is the first level of sleep which is characterised by the brain moving from drowsy alpha waves to the beginning of theta waves. Thoughts may begin to wander and be quite bizarre. The difference between this and other dream states is that in Stage 1, you are still virtually conscious. Indeed, this 'sleep' is so light that in sleep tests, during this stage 'patients often report having felt that they were awake'. A normal sleeper will only spend a few minutes in this stage before going deeper but an insomniac can spend most of the night in this 'half-sleep'.

Deep sleep, or 'slow wave' sleep is the deepest type of sleep in which no dreaming happens. It is also known as *delta* sleep because it is characterised by delta brain waves. This type of sleep is the most physically refreshing and when you have not had enough delta sleep, you may feel both physically and emotionally exhausted. If you often get up having dreamed vividly but feeling tense and unrefreshed, then you are probably not getting enough delta sleep.

REM sleep is the period of sleep in which we dream the most. REM stands for 'rapid eye movement'. This is because during REM sleep our eyes look around while dreaming, just as if we were wide awake. REM seems to be vital for our mental rejuvenation and general emotional well-being.

Together, these stages make up one full sleep cycle. During a normal night, a normal sleeper will go through several complete cycles and it is known that all three stages are essential for a refreshing night's sleep. One effect of sleeping medication is the disruption of this cycle. People awaking from a night of drugged sleep often feel unrefreshed, 'as if they hadn't slept at all'. This is in part due to not having had a complete night's sleep made up of all the essential stages.

The Effects and Side-Effects of Sleeping Pills

Hangover

Sleeping pills are known to reduce the amount of delta sleep obtained. This feeling of 'not having had enough sleep' associated with a lack of delta sleep makes the next day hangover all the more unpleasant. Almost every sleeping medication, including over-the-counter remedies, will leave you with a level of grogginess, thick-headedness, confusion or a 'spaced-out' feeling. These hangovers can be severe, affecting your reactions and ability to think, making driving or operating machinery very dangerous. In my experience, there is not a single conventional sleeping pill that does not cause some degree of hangover.

Depression and Mood

Sleeping pill hangovers often seem to be associated with a very low mood. Overall, the feeling of a sleeping pill hangover can be worse than the feeling after a sleepless night. Not only is delta sleep reduced, but many prescription drugs are known to reduce the time spent in REM sleep, which means that they interfere with mental recovery and emotional well-being. Bearing this in mind, it is not surprising that sleeping pills often cause daytime anxiety and depression.

Because insomnia can cause depression, it is often thought that insomnia medication may help to treat depression, and conversely, depression is sometimes thought to be the cause of insomnia. This results in anti-depressants such as Prozac being prescribed for insomnia patients, whether or not they have actually ever claimed to be depressed.

However, recent research suggests that both these assumptions are mistaken. An analysis of data of clinical trials submitted to the FDA found that patients taking sedative hypnotics were much *more* likely to develop depression. In fact, the popular drugs zolpidem, zaleplon and ezopiclone, more than *doubled* the risks of developing depression compared with those taking placebo pills[1]. Furthermore, studies have found that long-term users of sedative hypnotic drugs have a markedly raised suicide risk, particularly for men. The statistics showed that men who took a nightly sleeping pill actually had seven times the normal risk of suicide![2] Prescribing sleeping pills in the hope that this will relieve or prevent depression would appear to be a very unwise move indeed. Far from helping depressed patients, sleeping medication may be more likely to cause depression.

Addiction
Like any other addictive drug, almost all hypnotic sleeping pills have two main ways in which they can be addictive.
1. Firstly, if you have taken sleeping pills you will be familiar with how, after a time, the medication seems to stop

---

1   Kripke, D.F. 2007. 'Greater incidence of depression with hypnotic used than with placebo'. *BMC Psychiatry,* 21(7): 42
2   Kripke, D.F. et al. 2002. 'Mortality associated with sleep duration and insomnia'. *Arch Gen Psychiatry*, 59:131-136

working. As a result, higher and higher doses are needed to obtain the same effect. A common occurrence is that the drug eventually stops working altogether.

2. In addition, almost all sleeping pills have been shown to be physically addictive which means that withdrawal symptoms can be severe, even life-threatening. This happens even though the drug may have stopped having any beneficial effect. Withdrawal symptoms may include shakiness, anxiety, panic, palpitations, epileptic fits, increased insomnia and even death.

Between the 1960s and 1980s, most sleeping pills prescribed were benzodiazepines. But these highly addictive drugs came with a whole host of negative side-effects and some evidence suggests that benzodiazepine addiction can be more dangerous, and take longer to overcome, than heroin. However, while benzodiazepines are still often prescribed, these days you may be more likely to be given one of the newer 'non-benzodiazepines' including the 'Z-drugs' such as zopiclone (Imovane, Zimovane), ezopiclone (Lunesta), zolpidem (Ambien) and zaleplon (Sonata). If you have taken sleeping pills in the last ten years, then there is a good chance that you were prescribed one of these. Zopiclone is the drug most often prescribed for insomnia by the NHS. When non-benzodiazepines first appeared, they were hailed as having few or no addictive qualities or negative side-effects, and they were gratefully received by the market of eager insomniacs. Medical opinion of these drugs has now changed somewhat and it now appears that in some cases they can be as troublesome as the benzodiazepine drugs they were created to replace.

Benzodiazepines were responsible for the largest ever lawsuit against drug manufacturers in the United Kingdom, involving 14,000 patients. However, research suggests that the now ironically named 'non-benzodiazepines' are almost identical in effect and side-effect. In particular, research suggests that they have similarly addictive qualities.

A systematic review carried out in 2004 at the University of Liverpool compared the newer Z-drugs zaleplon, zolpidem and zopiclone with benzodiazepines and with each other. The factors compared in the review included: sleep onset latency, total sleep duration, number of awakenings, quality of sleep, adverse events, tolerance, rebound insomnia and daytime alertness. The report's conclusion may come as a surprise. It reports that regarding benzodiazepines and non-benzodiazepines "there are few clear, consistent differences between the drugs"[3]. It would appear that non-benzodiazepines such as zaleplon, zolpidem, zopiclone and ezopiclone may be no less addictive than the original benzodiazepines like Valium.

Performance

One of the most important reasons for needing sleep is to allow us to function well in the morning and go about our normal day's activities. Astonishingly, research shows that the use of sleeping pills does *not* increase your ability to function the next day. On the contrary, those taking sleeping pills will, *according to almost all clinical studies*, function *worse* the next day than those who miss a night's sleep![4]

'A person's hope and belief that a prescription sleeping pill will improve the person's function on the next day is consistently betrayed.'[5]

Tellingly, several studies show that people involved in car accidents are unusually likely to have taken sleeping pills[6,7]

---

3 Dundar, Y. et al. 2004. 'Comparative efficacy of newer hypnotic drugs for the short-term management of insomnia: a systematic review and meta-analysis.' *Hum Psychopharmacol.* 19(5): 305 – 22

4 Johnson, L.C. et al. 1982. 'Sedative-hypnotics and human performance.' *Psychopharmacology (Berlin).* 76:101 – 113)

5 Kripke, D.F. *The Dark Side of Sleeping Pills.*

6 Hemmelgarn, B. et al. 1997. 'Benzodiazepine use and the risk of motor vehicle crash in the elderly.' *JAMA.* 278:27 - 31.; Betts, T.A. et al. 1982.

Severe impairment can occur even after taking 'harmless' antihistamines prescribed for insomnia. Ucerax (hydroxine) is one such antihistamine, which is taken to help sleep. It is also prescribed for anxiety when the dosage can be as high as 50mg daily. Despite being billed as 'gentle', for some it appears to have a more powerful effect than any hypnotic. Personal and anecdotal evidence I have collected shows that even small doses of Ucerax can turn you into a walking 'zombie', unable to function properly at all and without the sense to realise that you are unfit to drive.

When it comes to next day performance, you may well be better off not having had any sleep than having had a full night of drugged sleep.

Rebound Insomnia

This refers to the temporary worsened insomnia which occurs when a patient attempts to give up a sleeping medication. Rebound insomnia is actually a side-effect of sleeping pill addiction and anyone embarking on a course of insomnia medication should bear in mind that *worse* is likely to come when the time comes to give up. Many people continue to take sleeping pills, not because they are benefiting in any way, but because they cannot stand the worsened insomnia which kicks in when they try to give up.

It is often once a medication has become almost ineffectual that a patient attempts to give it up. A study of flurazepam and triazolam showed that after five weeks of use, patients were sleeping no better than those receiving placebo[8]. The only reason that patients

'Effect of two hypnotic drugs on actual driving performance next morning.' *Br.Med.J,* 25:285 – 852

7   Barbone, F., McMahon, A.D., Davey, P.G. et al. 1998. 'Association of road-traffic accidents with benzodiazepine use'. *Lancet,* **352** (9137): 1331 – 6

8   Mitler, M.M. et al. 1984. 'Comparative hypnotic effects of flurazepam, triazolam, and placebo: a long-term simultaneous night-time and daytime study.' *J.Clin.Psychopharmacol,* 4:2 – 15.

so often continue to take medication after this point is because the rebound insomnia makes it simply too painful to stop. The patient becomes completely unable to sleep with or without pills. Sadly, they may become so desperate that a common response is to increase the dosage, even though the original good intention was to eliminate it altogether.

Non-Effectiveness – Sleeping Pills That Don't Make You Sleep

The desperate desire to simply 'fall asleep', to be unconscious can make sleeping pills a tempting prospect, even for those who know a bad day will follow. But believe it or not, in many 'successful' drug trials the increase in time spent sleeping is in the range of just 20 - 40 minutes! More astonishing are the results of trials on the non-benzodiazepine, zaleplon (Sonata). These showed that while it decreased sleep onset time by a paltry 11–12 minutes, it was *not* found to increase total sleep time![9] This means that while patients were falling asleep quicker, they were getting *less* sleep with Sonata than without it. Despite these results, zaleplon was licensed for sale and is still widely prescribed.

Early Waking

The odd effect mentioned in the last point – that some drugs decrease the time it takes to *fall* asleep while not increasing the time spent sleeping[10] – may have a pharmacological explanation. Many people taking triazolam (Halcion), zaleplon (Sonata), zolpidem (Ambien), zopiclone (Zimovane, Imovane) and eszopiclone (Lunesta) find that they fall asleep quite quickly but

---

9 Buscemi, N., Vandermeer, B., Friesen, C., et al. 2007. 'The efficacy and safety of drug treatments for chronic insomnia in adults: a meta-analysis of RCTs'. *J Gen Intern Med*, 22:1335 – 50

10 Kripke, D.F. *The Dark Side of Sleeping Pills*

wake very early in the morning, often in an agitated state, ranging from moderate unease to a mild panic attack. These medications are supposed to be ideal for those who find it hard to fall asleep, but who, once asleep, tend to stay asleep. Quite high doses are given to produce a sudden 'hit', but the drugs are very short acting, leaving the bloodstream completely after only a few hours. This is supposed to make them much less likely to cause a hangover the next day. The problem is that when the dose wears off in the early hours, the body can go into instant sudden withdrawal. Research suggests that it is this 'comedown' which wakes you up too early and causes anxiousness the next day, *not* the effect of the drug still in the bloodstream.

Mortality

Perhaps the most frightening fact about sleeping pills is that they increase your chances of *dying!* Sleeping pills may increase your chances of heart disease, serious illnesses, accidents and cancer.[11] The *mortality rate* refers to the percentage of people who have died in a given test group of people over a set time period. In people who regularly take sleeping pills this percentage is much higher. If you take a sleeping pill every night for six years you are 25% more likely to die than those who take none. Astonishingly, even those who take the occasional sleeping drug are 15% more likely to be dead in six years. Think about this: if you take a pill every night, in just six years you are 25% less likely to be here.

Summary of Effects

There are three ways in which a sleeping pill may be deemed effective.

---

11 Kripke, D.F. 'Evidence that new hypnotics cause cancer.' *BMC Psychiatry*, 7:42

1. It increases the time spent asleep.
2. It makes you fall asleep faster.
3. It increases next-day performance.

The sad truth is that no medication succeeds on all three counts. Most are effective in one way, but at the expense of one of the others. In addition, every sleeping pill comes with one or more of the following undesirable effects:

*   Decreases the time taken to fall asleep by a negligible amount
*   Does not increase the time spent asleep
*   May wake you earlier than if you had not taken medication
*   Does not improve your function the next day
*   Is highly addictive
*   Leaves you with an unpleasant hangover
*   Increases your chances of developing serious illness, such as cancer and heart disease
*   Causes depression and anxiety
*   Increases your chances of dying by 25%
*   Causes rebound insomnia
*   Is not as effective as behavioural treatment for the treatment of insomnia

Treating long-term chronic insomnia with hypnotic sleeping pills is somewhat like treating depression with cocaine. When sleeping pills are prescribed, the *symptom* of 'being awake' is treated completely in isolation, with no regard for the cause of the problem or the side-effects of the treatment. In both cases, the patient may become addicted. Both sleeping pills and cocaine come with a host of horrible side-effects and with prolonged use, whatever positive effect they may have diminishes. The ideal outcome in both cases is that a person quickly comes to realise that the costs outweigh the benefits, and is able to stop before a real problem sets in. Therefore it is not an exaggeration to say that with cocaine and sleeping pills, the effect and outcome are almost identical. There would be an outcry if doctors started prescribing cocaine to depressives, but the prescribing of sleeping medication for insomniacs is standard practice.

The Truth about Sleeping Pill Research – Who Pays for it?

So, if these drugs really have so many disadvantages and side-effects, why are they ever licensed for sale? It is a little-known fact that almost all research into sleeping pills is not independent but is funded by drug companies. In a recent article published in The Journal of Clinical Sleep Medicine[12], details were given of a systematic review of the medical literature concerning insomnia drugs. It found that over 90% of randomised controlled trials of drug treatments of insomnia are sponsored by the pharmaceutical industry itself. This means that there was almost no independent research at all. The most worrying evidence given in the article was that industry-sponsored drug trials were more than *3½ times more likely* to deem a drug effective than non-industry sponsored trials.

Some drugs were pronounced successful and effective and are now been currently prescribed even though the test results were less than satisfactory. An increase of 11 – 12 minutes' sleep has been enough for trials to be hailed as successful and consequently for a drug to be licensed for sale. Moreover, according to the review, the positive effects of a particular medication were overemphasised in the medical literature. For example, success might be reported with regard to sleep onset time, but with no discussion of associated adverse effects, such as significant increased levels of infection, cancers and increased mortality. According to the review

---

12 Kripke, D.F. 2007. 'Who Should Sponsor Sleep Disorders Pharmaceutical Trials?,' *J Clin Sleep Med.* 3(7): 671 – 673

'major hypnotic trials are needed to more carefully study potential adverse effects of hypnotics such as daytime impairment, infection, cancer, and death and the resultant balance of benefits and risks.'

The Extraordinary Placebo Effect of Sleeping Pills

A large study[13] was carried out on a group of chronic insomniacs who had also been succesfully taking benzodiazepines for an average of 13 years.The volunteers were randomly assigned to receive either Dalmane, midazolam, or to receive inactive placebo pills. Remarkably, after nine to 14 days of administration, there was no statistically-reliable increase at all in the sleep of the patients taking Dalmane or midazolam as compared with those receiving placebo. The patients had already become tolerant to the medication. Furthermore, by 14 days, both drugs were making next day performance significantly worse. Astonishingly, the patients themselves said that they thought the medication was good and that it was helping them, even when objective tests showed that the medications were making them worse.

But more interesting than this is that part of the reason that the sleeping pills showed no significant benefit was that the placebo group had also improved. Most tellingly, even the group receiving placebo reported that they rated the medication they had been given highly and would be happy to use it again. The group receiving either Dalmane or midazolam rated their pill slightly more highly than the placebo group, even although the active drugs were worse for the patients than the placebo.

---

13 Kripke, , D.F. et al. 1990. 'Sleep evaluation in chronic insomniacs during 14-day use of flurazepam and midazolam.' *J.Clin.Psychopharmacol.* 10(Supplement 4):32S – 43S.

'These patients were self-deceived about the value of the medication, almost deluded, thinking the medicines made them better when they actually made them worse.'[14]

The placebo effect is well-known with all drugs but when dealing with insomnia, which is so powerfully affected by suggestion and belief, this effect may be even greater.

Some Worrying Facts about Sleeping Pill Prescription

In a large study done in the US, around a third of people who regularly took sleeping pills reported *never having had insomnia.* A more worrying statistic concerns long-term chronic insomniacs. The rationale behind sleeping pills is that medication can be beneficial to people with short-term insomnia in helping to normalise sleeping patterns. However, when we look at patterns of prescription, a more complicated story emerges. While most people will only take a dozen or so doses in any one year, chronic users will take many more. It is to these chronic insomniacs, and not to the occasional sufferers, that most of the drugs are prescribed. The truth is that 65% of sleeping pills currently being taken are prescribed, not to short-term users, but to those who have been taking them every night for five years! This appalling statistic shows that the multi-million pound sleeping pill industry is

'profiting primarily from chronic users who have become habituated or physically addicted to these medicines'[15]

---

14 Kripke, D.F. *The Dark Side of Sleeping Pills,* op. cit.

15 Kripke, D.F. Ibid.

Mosquitoes – a case in point

The power of the drug companies over medical 'knowledge' and treatment should not be underestimated. I recently had a vivid personal illustration of this: I have suffered terribly with mosquitoes whenever I have spent time in a hot country. I have lost count of how many creams, antihistamines and cortisones I have been prescribed and sold by doctors and pharmacists over the decades. Only last year I was told of an old 'folk remedy' which involves applying very hot wet towels to the bites themselves. The theory is that the body can only make a certain amount of histamine in any ten hour period. By applying the hot cloth, all the histamine in that part of the body rushes to the skin at once. The body will then take up to ten hours to replenish its histamine levels, at which point the itch will start again. It works like magic! But the astonishing thing is that no medical professional ever knew of this free remedy ... or, at least in the 40 years of my life, none has ever *told* me of this free remedy! After a lifetime of suffering on almost every holiday, and almost every summer, even in England, and after countless visits to the doctor and pharmacist, and countless amounts spent on remedies, I discovered a free and safe way to completely cure the itching from mosquito bites. And in all those years, not *one* healthcare professional in any country had done anything other than prescribe and sell me utterly useless pharmaceuticals. So folks, there is a safe, easy, virtually free and highly effective remedy for mosquito bite itching out there and no doctor will ever tell you about it!

The Secret No Doctor Will Tell You –
Why Sleeping Pills Can Cause Insomnia

Most of these negative aspects of sleeping medication are well known. But besides all these well-documented 'medical' dangers of sleeping pills, perhaps a greater concern are the psychological and emotional side-effects of taking sleeping drugs. The remarkable but incontrovertible fact is:

Sleeping pills can make insomnia worse.

Note that this is a completely separate issue to the rebound insomnia which usually occurs when a person tries to give up. Because insomnia is treated by doctors as a medical condition, little time and consideration is given over to the emotional and psychological impact on beliefs about sleep. Consider, for a moment, the message implicit in the prescribing of a sleeping pill – *'this pill will make you sleep.'*

In the short term, this thought can be comforting. Because responsibility is taken away, you may stop worrying enough to fall asleep. No one tells us about the unacknowledged inherent danger in this – that in giving up responsibility, you give up your *power*. If you need a pill to make you sleep then the implication is that you must be unable to sleep on your own. This means that when you take a sleeping pill, any success will be attributed to the medication. The result is that you come to trust more and more in the drug and less and less in yourself until, eventually, you have lost *all* belief and trust in your own ability to sleep. When your self-belief becomes completely eroded natural, effortless sleep then becomes a distant memory.

If sleeping pills always came with some form of counselling, or guidelines which would work on increasing your own trust in yourself, then perhaps their effect would be more beneficial. Instead, when insomnia patients are prescribed medication, they are given a temporary, and inherently harmful, crutch with no suggestion of how to go about overcoming their underlying problem. This is why, in addition to any physically addictive qualities, *all* sleeping medications can be so incredibly habit-forming. The truth is that

**Any artificial crutch
will decrease your confidence
in your own ability to sleep.**

This is the main reason why sleeping tablets can *never* really cure insomnia. The problem will still always be there, hiding under the surface and waiting to pop out again as soon as the medication is stopped, or stops working, often in a much more virulent form than before. This is why *sleeping pills can actually make insomnia worse.*

The Effortless Sleep Method necessarily uses no drugs whatsoever. Its aim is to restore a person's normal ability to sleep naturally and unaided – *there is not a single drug available that can do this.*

CHAPTER FOUR

Sleep Restriction Therapy
When Good Sleep Hygiene Rules Go Bad!

Sleep Restriction Therapy (often abbreviated to SR) is the standard and perhaps most widely used non-drug treatment for insomnia in sleep clinics across the UK, Europe and the US. It is one of the few non-drug treatments available on the NHS. If you are lucky enough to be referred to a sleep specialist, you may be unlucky enough to be advised to embark on a sleep restriction programme. There are some interesting books written on the subject including the classic *Desperately Seeking Snoozing,* by John Wiedman[16].

At first sight, Sleep Restriction Therapy appears simply as a more hardline version of sleep hygiene – a set of common-sense guidelines, which instil good habits, lay a foundation for natural sleep to occur and can help to normalise sleeping patterns. Because it is sometimes assumed that their basic premises for working are the same, many insomniacs can be resistant to any form of 'sleep rule'. This is a big mistake. Later in the book I will show that while good sleep hygiene is not always enough to cure an established problem, without it it can be near-impossible to overcome insomnia. The mechanism by which SR works is actually quite different. Through absolute adherence to a set of very strict rules

---

16 I am mentioned in this 1997 book. Wiedman included online postings from various insomniacs and I was one of them. Here is proof of the longevity of my problem!

SR actually induces a state of extreme sleep deprivation. The idea is to drastically limit the time spent in bed, although advice about exactly how long this time should be varies. Some recommend just enough sleep to allow you to function, *not* enough to feel good, happy and refreshed, but *just* enough so that you can survive the next day. For most people this is between five and six hours. Other advocates of SR insist that you should limit the time spent in bed to just that amount of sleep you are currently getting. So if you are getting only four hours per night, you should only stay in bed for four hours.

So, for example, if you are limiting your time to five hours in bed, and you need to get up at 6.30am for work, you must not go to bed until 1.30am. If you have not fallen asleep within 15 – 20 minutes of lying down then you *must* get up, go to another room, and only return to bed when you are sleepy. If still you do not fall asleep within 20 minutes then you must once again get up and stay up until you feel sleepy. This process should be repeated, all night if necessary, until you fall asleep. And, no matter how little or how much you have slept, you *must* still get up 6.30am, even if you have been in and out of bed ten times in the night and have not slept at all. During the day, naps are strictly forbidden and you must not close your eyes to sleep until bedtime at 1.30 the next night.

The theory behind SR is straightforward: by severely limiting the time spent in bed, this regime *forces* you to sleep. The idea is that at some point, even the most chronic insomniac will be so exhausted they will be unable to fight the sleep instinct. In a state of such sleep deprivation, exhaustion overrides the ability to stay awake and, eventually, you will sleep. Once a regular pattern has been established of solid sleeping on this tiny amount, the time spent in bed can be increased *slowly* in, perhaps, 15-minute increments.

Sound reasonable? Try it!

Be warned: you will need limitless motivation and superhuman powers of discipline to manage a sleep restriction programme. These rules can be near-impossible to stick to. Many people find SR unacceptably strict and harsh, and for some (including me), it is little short of torture.

Just as an example, imagine the following scenario. This is typical of the experiences of those who have written to me disillusioned by SR. Suppose you have started a Sleep Restriction Programme and have set your ration of sleep to five hours per night. One week in, you have stuck to the rule of spending only five hours in bed per night. On most nights you have not managed to fall asleep within thirty minutes and so have had to get up a few times. In other words, you have not yet managed to get a full five hours of sleep. Now imagine that one night you can't bring yourself to get out of bed after 20 minutes of lying awake. Perhaps it is winter and the heating is off and the thought of getting up into the freezing night is just too unpleasant. Because of this, you stay in bed. You sleep badly, partly because you are worried that by not sticking to the rules you may have affected the programme. At 6.30am the alarm goes off and you manage to get up and drag yourself to work. Somehow you manage to struggle through the day in a state of extreme sleep deprivation. Finally, it is 1.30am and time for bed. But because of last night's rule breaking, you are tense and worried. Perhaps this slip-up will affect your ability to sleep tonight? Understandably, you do not manage to fall asleep within 20 minutes and so have to get up and spend some of your precious rest time out of bed. Back in bed at 3.30am, it's only three hours now until you have to get up!

Finally, at 4am, you fall into a blissful, delicious sleep. Your mind and body relax gratefully with relief. Sweet dreams turn to deep delta sleep and you *rest,* finally. But then … horror of horrors! At 6.30am your alarm goes off and you are violently awakened from the best sleep you have had in weeks. This is horrific! Getting up having not slept is bad enough, but getting up having slept *a little* is even worse! It is unbearable. The desire to sleep is so strong it is torment to resist. To make matters worse, it is Saturday and there is no added motivation to get up for work. You turn the alarm off and lie there, sleep still heavy on you, creeping back, tempting you. You could be back asleep within seconds if you do not get up right now. You know you should get up, you know that the programme will be undermined if you don't drag yourself up right *now*. But hey, surely you need this sleep, don't you? It is Saturday after all. It might do you some good, in fact, it might take the pressure off a bit and just another half an hour will still be less than … too late. You give in to the overpowering sleep instinct and wake up three hours later, well-rested and refreshed.

But rather than feeling motivated and encouraged by this good night's sleep, there is only disappointment that you have sabotaged the programme. You have failed, in fact. You may feel physically good today, but your hopes and chances of sleeping this next night are greatly diminished, making you miserable and hopeless.

The same is true if you inadvertently (or semi-intentionally) nod off coming home from work on the train, or at 6pm after dinner in front of the television. If you stay awake for 19 hours a day, the chances of avoiding an accidental nap are so small as to be near-impossible. When that lovely sleepy feeling comes over you on the train, it takes unimaginable willpower to resist and the most frustrating thing is, every such nap or oversleep is a set-back on the SR programme.

To explain why, you need to understand the mechanism by which the programme works: SR works by *inducing sleep deprivation*. The upshot is that the more sleep you get, the more the effect of sleep deprivation is weakened. The amount of sleep must be increased in small increments, allowing patterns *gradually* to become normalised. So any *sudden* disruption to the programme, any accidental nap or oversleep, means that the sleep deprivation effect is wiped out. The consequence of this is that because you are *not* sleep deprived, there is no other means by which the programme can work, *and so there is no other means by which you can sleep*. After all, this programme works through inducing sleep deprivation and even a short nap can be quite refreshing, making you less sleep-deprived than you might be. The system is supposed to remove the pressure to sleep, by insisting that you stay awake for such long periods. But in reality, the pressure is only increased every time one of these *inevitable* slip-ups happens. Paradoxically, getting a *full night's sleep* early on in the programme is not a cause for celebration. On the contrary, it means beginning all over again; it means failure.

It is heartbreaking to receive messages from desperate people who have 'slipped off the wagon', who have given up on SR because they just couldn't stand it, or who have bent the rules and now wonder why it isn't working any more. In my experience, far from increasing your confidence, SR just sets you up to fail. It promises to help the most desperate of insomniacs and then punishes them when they are unable to stick to its barbaric rules. Sleep Restriction Therapy is cruel and it is unworkable. Try it, if you want; I wouldn't prescribe it to my worst enemy.

Sleep Restriction Therapy as a Crutch

You may find forum posts or internet messages from some people who swear that SR has helped them. Apparently, for some, SR can encourage a regular pattern of sleep. But even for these people who claim success with SR, can it give the sort of long term, confident, sure sleep that the Effortless Sleep System does? Does it give you real belief that you can sleep, that you are *better*?

The reason why SR works for some people may have little to do with the restriction itself. It may well work because a person *believes* it will work. Sticking to the rules gives a feeling of trust, as responsibility is handed over to the programme itself. Drug therapy and Sleep Restriction Therapy thus have one thing in common – both act as an external, artificial aid to sleep.

Because both SR and drug therapy are external and artificial, the hardcore insomniac's mind can always find a reason to start doubting, or a flaw to exploit. SR often seems to work in the short term but if you read the online message boards, you will often find SR patients saying 'I could sleep when in bed for six hours but as soon as I increased it to six and a quarter my insomnia returned'. This happens because the increase of the extra time in bed allowed doubt to creep in. Like pills, the suggestion is that it is the SR which *makes* you sleep. Without any confidence in your own abilities to sleep, you become utterly dependent upon the method, with no idea of how to go it alone.

So, perhaps the biggest problems with both drugs and SR is that there is no suggestion that it is *you* who is able to sleep, that it is *you* who is letting sleep happen. The assumption is that the pills, or the strict regime, is *making* you sleep. Just like the poor people addicted to sleeping pills, SR becomes an addiction and just like sleeping pills, one night without it means a return of insomnia. Just like sleeping tablets, SR is a habit which will need to be kicked. At some point you are going to have to start believing, stop obsessing, and move on.

In other words, you are going to have to come to realisations similar to those proposed in this book. At some point you will have to end up here – dealing with your own thoughts, attitudes, behaviours and beliefs about insomnia. Until you change your thoughts about insomnia, until you have genuine confidence in your own ability to sleep unaided, there will always be a lurking fear that one day the problem will return. If you do not also attend to any underlying, self-sabotaging, reinforcing beliefs and behaviours, these will either prevent the programme from working for you, or will remain lurking, ready to cause a relapse at the first slip-up.

Tellingly, according to one online sleep restriction programme "insomnia is likely to recur again at some point". And if it lasts more than a few nights, the advice is to "immediately implement

Sleep Restriction again". No sleep specialist can claim real success in a therapy or plan and then say that the problem is *likely* to recur at some point.

If you do not have absolute faith that your insomnia is beaten this doubt alone will stop you from truly recovering. You need nothing short of complete confidence that chronic insomnia will never return in its previous form. This is the kind of permanent change which the Effortless Sleep Method is designed to create and is the kind of change which can never take place by using drugs, or SR, or any other external therapy.

...3...

PRELIMINARIES AND PHILOSOPHY

CHAPTER FIVE

The Philosophy Behind
The Effortless Sleep Method

Now that you have heard the reasons why conventional means are so often ineffective in the battle against insomnia, you are probably wondering what is different about this system. This method will be quite unlike any other kind of sleeping aid you will have come across before. I am going to give you something altogether more reliable, more lasting, more natural than an artificial crutch – nothing less than the power and confidence to sleep naturally and unaided.

Every external 'cure', including drugs and SR, must eventually become a crutch. However, the funny thing is:

We all use crutches to fall asleep!

The truth is that there is nothing *intrinsically* wrong with having a crutch to help you sleep. For example, one woman who wrote to me is unable to sleep without earplugs. She developed this habit years ago when some thoughtless neighbours were keeping her up all night, and decades later she is unable to sleep without them. But because earplugs have no side-effects, are easily worn no matter where she is sleeping, and are readily available in every country in the world, it doesn't much matter whether she wears them every night for the rest of her life. She tells me that when she puts in her earplugs it is like escaping into her own secret, silent little sanctuary where she can shut out the outside world. A crutch like this is no more than a safety net, just like a child's teddy bear or comfort blanket. If there were a pill or aid that would help you sleep every single night and that you became utterly dependent on, even though you couldn't sleep without it, there really would be no problem as long as there were no harmful side-effects *and* it was completely reliable. The problem is that there are very few, if any, external sleeping aids which are like this. To start with, there is no external sleep aid which works for everybody. Just because earplugs or lavender pillows help one person does not mean that they will help the next. And, of course, many external crutches come with negative side-effects of their own. But the greatest problem with *external,* artificial crutches such as sleeping pills and sleep restriction therapies is that eventually they are liable to let you down. While some may be intrinsically harmless, none can be 100% reliable when there is always the danger that the aid will be unavailable one night, or that doubt will creep in. When this happens, because there is no self-belief left in place of the now worthless safety net, you will have no idea of how to go it alone. So if you rely on an artificial crutch or safety net, you are playing a dangerous game; sooner or later, that crutch could let you down and you will be cast adrift with nothing to comfort you but the belief that you cannot sleep unaided … In fact, there is only one safety net really worth having, one which, once in place, will *never* let you down.

The Best Type of Safety Net

There is really no need to use a faulty, harmful, unreliable, or unpleasant safety net such as Sleep Restriction or pills. Instead, imagine if your safety net were the *belief* that you could actually sleep! Sound crazy? Not when you consider this: the unconscious belief in the ability to sleep effortlessly is the safety net that every normal sleeper relies upon and relaxes into every night. A safety net is just something that you trust unconditionally. It is something you do not doubt or think about. Good sleepers don't even think about whether they can sleep – they just *trust* that they can. In fact, the only reason anyone ever falls asleep is because of *trust,* either in themselves or in something external, like a pill or relaxation tape. So, you see, we all use a safety net to fall asleep.

Your safety net is probably full of holes, or may even be completely missing. If there is no safety net, there is no trust, and no belief. It should thus come as no surprise that your body will not allow you to 'fall' into sleep. But we are going to help you to weave a new net, a strong net, one that you can relax into every night, which will *never* let you down. To begin with this will take the form of a conscious and tentative belief. But over time, the belief will become ingrained, become unconscious, become complete *trust* just like the very best sleepers. When this happens, you will have no more need for sleeping aids; you will have the ultimate sleeping aid at your disposal every night and everywhere you go.

**This whole method is about creating
an altogether different type of crutch, the best kind,
a safety net in the form of a belief that you can sleep.**

- CHAPTER SIX -

Preliminaries

To give this programme the very best chance of working for you, you will need to read the information in this chapter very carefully. The first part contains common-sense instructions on how to approach the programme. The remainder explains the background assumptions on which this method is based. It is particularly important that you read and carefully digest the advice in this chapter before going *near* the sections on the cure itself. All these preliminaries need to be read *and completely accepted* if you are to get the full benefit from the Effortless Sleep Method.

You Will Need to be Really, Really Honest with Yourself

This programme involves taking a good look at yourself, your thoughts and your behaviours. It is essential that you take complete responsibility for both your problem and your recovery and this will not be possible if you start out by deceiving or kidding yourself in some respect. For example, if you read that 'most long term insomniacs usually make the mistake of …', you will need to be really honest with yourself about whether this applies to you. The next chapter contains a description of some of the most common mistakes that insomniacs tend to make. If you claim never to exhibit any of these behaviours then you will probably need to look a bit harder. The truth is that someone who makes none of these mistakes is very unlikely to have a problem sleeping!

If you really want to be over this problem then, from this point on, you need to be *completely* honest with yourself regarding your sleep behaviour.

Your Problem is Not Special

Do you think one of the following statements is true of you?

My problem is not the same as these others I read about.
The type of person I am means sleep remedies don't work on me.
I think the things you have said so far don't apply to me.
Nothing works for me.
I don't sleep like normal people.
I have a broken sleep mechanism.
My problem is different.
I'm different.

I have some news for you. *None* of the above statements is true, of you or of anyone else! If you think that your problem is different, worse or that there will never be a cure for your particular situation, then think again. I suffered for 15 miserable years, believing I was somehow different, that I had a 'faulty switch'. And it was *this feeling*, this belief that 'my problem was different' that stopped me accepting a lot of what is true about the right way to treat insomnia.

There is no such thing as a 'broken sleep mechanism' or a 'faulty sleep response' or any other such thing. No one is physically or psychologically *unable* to sleep. In fact, we are all born with the same natural sleeping response. But we also have the ability to fight this instinct to prevent us from falling asleep in times of danger. This means that sleep is a delicate thing and for some, poor sleep habits and negative beliefs are enough to override the falling asleep response. The truth is that falling asleep is not about *doing* something, like taking a pill. It's about *not* doing something. Take away those faulty habits and beliefs and sleep happens automatically. There really is nothing else to 'fix'. When you stop doing the things which prevent you from sleeping, *you will sleep*.

Don't Look For Ways to Make Me Wrong

Which of the following statements apply to you?

I need medical/scientific proof that something will work.
I need something to 'sound right' before I can accept it.
I've tried something similar and it didn't help.
This doesn't sound right to me.
I'm very hard to convince.
I'll give this a go only if I like the sound of it.
Who are you to tell me what to do?

Do you have an inquiring, sceptical mind? Research shows that chronic insomniacs are usually of well-above average intelligence. This probably explains why they seem to have an answer for everything, a counterexample for every example they hear, and why they can pick the holes in any argument, or any system, or any remedy. It's amazing really, the way that insomniacs always seem to know best with regard to their problem. It's even more surprising that, given that they know best, they often go on to continue suffering for decades! It's a gift to be intelligent, it's wonderful that you can be right so often, isn't it? Now answer the following question:

Is it more important to you to get over your insomnia, or to be right?

For *once* your intelligence is not going to be an asset. Close down that intelligent, questioning mind and trust like an ignorant, innocent child. Remember: ignorant, innocent children sleep *effortlessly* without questioning how or why. Just trust, be honest with yourself, follow the advice and let the programme work its magic. You are about to be shown the *only* way to turn your problem around. Don't find ways to disagree, don't find ways to make it wrong, don't look for ways in which your problem is different. Don't say 'but ..., but ..., but ...,' *listen and believe!* It's only when I stopped finding ways to disagree, stopped believing that there was something different and unique about my problem that I even *began* to recover.

If you find some of the advice difficult to accept, then *give it the benefit of the doubt*! What's the worst that can happen? Follow it, to the letter, and *then* decide to agree or disagree with the approach.

If you concentrate on finding ways to argue with the programme, or prove me wrong, or if you decide from the off that 'this won't work' or 'I've done things like that before, I can skip that bit', if any or all of the above are true for you then be warned, the Effortless Sleep Method will not help you and you will be back on your own.

There is a Mental and a Behavioural Aspect to Chronic Insomnia

For people with a long-term or established problem there are always two aspects to their insomnia – psychological and behavioural. Most chronic insomniacs find that the more they worry about sleep, the worse their problem becomes. Even if your problem is very recent or intermittent, you will know that worrying about sleep makes the problem worse. Many find that reading about someone else's problem, or learning about a new potential threat to sleep can make theirs worse. On the other hand, no matter how many different experiments and remedies and combinations they try, none of them *ever* seem to work. Stop and think about this a moment because there is something incredible to be learned here: the problem seems to get worse at the drop of a hat yet seems impossible to improve. How can this be? What sort of an illness is it that can get instantly worse simply because of something you hear? The answer is very simple:

Chronic insomnia is largely a mental problem

If your sleep habits and routines are good then your insomnia must have a psychological basis. Ironically, while the long-term insomniac will allow the merest suggestion to worsen their problem, when it comes to finding a solution, they will almost always look to external, physical methods such as drugs to alleviate the problem. Sadly, this is about as effective as trying to fix a burst pipe by thinking about it.

If your insomnia is a mental problem, then it has a mental solution.

In truth, the mechanics of insomnia reveal its cure. If chronic insomnia is caused by faulty thinking and negative beliefs, it can only be changed by attending to those thoughts, not by taking a drug, or using fans, magnets, special pillows, lavender bags or having a special crystal next to your bed!

It is astonishing that so few insomniacs know or accept this, especially after so many years of watching the suggestion → fear → worsening insomnia dynamic in process. But don't be surprised if this is the first time you have realised this or are still finding it difficult to believe: it took me 15 years to accept where the remedy to my insomnia lay.

But insomnia is not a problem which resides *only* in the mind. A few nights of insomnia become a chronic problem, not just because of faulty beliefs about sleep, but due to a whole host of contributing behaviours which *reinforce* your insomnia, keeping the problem firmly in place. Some of these behaviours are related to your sleeping and going-to-bed habits and for those with a recent problem, attending to these bed-related aspects will be all it takes to recover. The other behaviours are more subtle and insidious and you are unlikely to have heard of them. These behaviours are the most harmful and make the negative beliefs very difficult to change independently.

This programme will show you that by attending to both sets of negative behaviours you will find it much easier to improve your sleep patterns than if you concentrated on the beliefs alone. Attempting to break a long-held belief, or to force a new one, is very difficult. But this process is made much easier if at the same time we work on the much easier task of changing the *behaviours.* In this way we can move from mere wishful thinking to permanent, true beliefs, supported by new, positive behaviours.

If You Follow These Instructions You Will Recover

If you follow these guidelines you will beat your insomnia naturally,
... and forever.

A word of warning: re-read the sentence above in italics.

If you follow these guidelines you will beat your insomnia naturally,
... and forever.

The most important word in this statement is *if.* Because the one reason that this programme may not work for you is *if* you don't follow it.

All you need to do at the moment, is to entertain the possibility that this approach *works.* It worked for me, it worked for my team, and it will work for you. Sometimes people write to me, saying the programme hasn't helped them. Whenever I investigate I find it has always been for the same reason: *without exception* it is because they haven't followed the instructions.

The Two Negative Principles of the Mind

1. We tend to focus on the negative

It is strange but true that most human beings tend to focus chronically on *what they do not want*. It can be difficult to spot this tendency in yourself, especially if you do not consider yourself to be a particularly negative person. But just try observing yourself for a few days. See how much of your thinking time is spent focussed on what is wrong with your life. Then notice how little time you spend even *noticing* the good things, let alone celebrating them. How often do you appreciate the little things which turn out well – 'this coffee is just right', 'this sofa is comfy', 'my husband always remembers to put the seat down'! We usually don't even notice how often things go well for us and completely take for granted all the good in our lives. On the other hand, *negative* things, however small, tend to get focussed and remarked upon – 'this coffee is too strong', 'this sofa needs cleaning', 'my husband has left the towel on the floor *again'*. Even happy and positive people will tend to spend much of their time working out which aspects of their life need to be changed or improved. Judging things to be unsatisfactory can occasionally have the positive effect of inspiring change and improvement. But for insomniacs, it is incredibly destructive to be continually focusing on the negative. If, for example, they had one bad night's sleep along with three or four good ones, most insomniacs would focus on the *one* bad night! Not only does this give an inaccurate and exaggerated picture of the problem, it can actually worsen it.

2. What we focus on gets bigger

We all know what it is like to obsess about a particular aspect of our lives with which we are less than happy. It may be a lost relationship, a weight problem or an annoying colleague. The more time that is spent thinking about and around the issue, turning it upside down and back to front, examining it, considering its effect, the more important it seems to become. It then seems to grow out of all proportion and assume a life of its own and can take over our thinking, even though those around us may tell us we are overreacting, that we shouldn't let such a thing bother us so much.

But notice what happens when something comes along to forcibly take your mind off this particular issue, be it something novel and exciting or a *new* problem. What was previously the dominant thought in your life suddenly becomes unimportant, irrelevant even. You start a new and exciting relationship and suddenly the annoying colleague, the one who was causing you to consider leaving your job, becomes insignificant. You decide to move house and suddenly the latest shocking government scandal which had been dominating your life is forgotten.

But when nothing comes along to take our minds off our problems, we may continue to focus on them intently, increasing their severity. The fact is that whatever you focus on will grow and come to dominate your thoughts and your life. But very few people realise that the opposite is also true – focus on the good things in life and they become magnified in the same way. In fact, if you can cultivate a habit of focussing on whatever *good* there is in your life, this can make the difference between enjoying one's life and not.

You should keep these two vital points in mind as you read this book. *We tend to focus on what we do not want* and *what we focus on tends to get bigger.* All of us, insomniac or not, could benefit from incorporating these beliefs into our lives. If all you took away from this course was a full understanding of these two principles then this alone could have an astounding effect on your sleep and the quality of your life. These two psychological principles largely explain why insomnia can persist for such a long time. In a nutshell, insomniacs tend to focus on how *bad* their problem is, thinking and talking about the *worst* nights while often completely ignoring and taking for granted the really *good* nights. But the details are subtler. Read on, you are about to find out the finer details of how insomnia occurs in the first place, and why it can turn chronic so easily.

...4...

THE MAKING
OF A MONSTER

CHAPTER SEVEN

Why Insomnia Occurs

The Two Main Types of Insomnia

Transient insomnia refers to what most people experience at some point and lasts a few days or a few weeks. If you find it impossible to sleep on Sunday nights, or before an important event, or you are experiencing a 'bad patch' of sleep, perhaps because you are under particular stress, then you have *transient* insomnia. You may have had these bad patches several times in your life and have had no way of dealing with the problem other than using prescription drugs or over-the-counter remedies.

Chronic insomnia. If, on the other hand, you have been troubled by poor sleep for many years, if your 'bad patches' seem to outweigh your 'good patches', and if you regularly spend nights getting no more than a few hours' sleep, if it has become a major problem in your life, then you are a *chronic* insomniac. Chronic insomniacs typically become 'obsessed' by their problem and have usually tried countless prescription medicines and alternative remedies. They often report that 'nothing works' for them.

Within either of these divisions, people fall into two more groups. Those who find it difficult to fall asleep in the first place – *sleep onset* insomniacs and those who fall asleep quite quickly but who wake too early and find it impossible to get back to sleep – *sleep maintenance* insomniacs. You may not know (or care) which category or subcategory of insomniac you fall into. Happily, it makes no difference which label you might feel like applying to your particular sleeping problem – the system explained in this book is a 'one size fits all' cure, whether you have been suffering for two weeks or 20 years. Whichever of these sleep problems you have, the system laid out in this programme will have a profoundly beneficial effect on your sleep.

Short-term, transient insomnia usually occurs either during a period of extreme stress, or as a result of accidental poor sleeping habits. Often, these two things go together. This is because a common response to a missed night of sleep through stress is to lie in, or try to take naps during the day, thus creating poor sleeping patterns. Usually, transient insomnia rights itself and almost every person has experienced a run of insomnia at some point in his or her life. But for some people, these bouts of insomnia become more and more frequent, even becoming the norm, and runs of good nights of sleep become the exception. Some people even get to a stage where they cannot remember the last time they had a really good period of sleep.

The scary truth is that all chronic insomniacs started out as transient insomniacs and there is always a danger that any short spell of sleeplessness could turn into a more serious problem. Why does this happen? And why does insomnia sometimes remain long after the original stress or cause has disappeared or even been forgotten? One of the greatest frustrations for a chronic insomniac is in trying to work out why *their* insomnia lasts for years while others seem able to get over a bad patch of sleep very quickly, often by using a simple remedy such as a relaxation CD. It is hardly surprising that

chronic insomniacs often feel 'broken' or different.

This next section is vital to the programme. It shows in great detail the way that a mild patch of poor sleep can become chronic. If you are new to insomnia, this information will be invaluable in preventing your problem from becoming worse. If, on the other hand, your problem is already chronic, understanding this process will be *essential* to your recovery. Indeed, without an understanding of the way that a few missed nights can become (and remain) a life-long problem, it is my belief that a chronic insomniac may *never* recover. So before tackling your problem head-on, we must fully examine the psychology of insomnia.

The theory behind my approach is that insomnia is not just about sleep; it encroaches into one's whole life. As such, we *must* take a holistic approach, attending to thoughts and beliefs about sleep, and to habits and behaviours which create and reinforce the problem. In order to do this, the next chapter will focus on the various ways in which we create and maintain the problem, in order that these may be addressed and dealt with. This may seem unnecessarily negative but bear with it; reading this chapter will do nothing to make your problem worse. Through learning about the classic mistakes that insomniacs make, you will see the way we give life to insomnia, how it arises and why it gets so much worse in some people. Understanding these things in a general way will allow you to go on to discover the specific ways in which you do similar things in your own life. Only then will you be in a position to begin the process of getting your life back.

There are 13 mistakes which people unwittingly make along the road to insomnia. Be honest: how many of these are you guilty of?

CHAPTER EIGHT

A Recipe for Insomnia: How to Make a Monster in 13 Easy Mistakes

Mistake 1:
SPENDING TOO LONG IN BED

Insomnia does not always begin during a period of stress, as is often assumed. Very often, insomnia begins during a period when one is simply spending longer than usual in bed. Students, the self-employed and unemployed all frequently lie in until very late in the morning, and very often, times such as these are the beginning of a long problem.

This is compounded by the fact that a natural early response to a bout of insomnia is either to go to bed earlier, before you are even sleepy, or to try to 'catch up' by lying in bed for as long as possible. A very common mistake is to lounge around in bed in the morning even when you aren't sleeping, creating a mental association of being in bed with being awake. After a really poor night, it can be doubly hard to drag oneself out of bed at a good hour, and when fatigued and miserable it can seem easier to hide away in bed than to get up and face the day.

Often when you go to bed the night after a long lie-in, you may not be particularly tired when you lie down, with the result that it takes hours to fall asleep. To add to this, spending too long in bed means that your sleep becomes lighter and of poorer quality. If you feel exhausted even if you have slept for many hours, then there is a good chance that you are spending far too long in bed.

Try to remember:
>**If you are spending more time in bed**
>**than you did before your insomnia started,**
>**then this is almost certainly a key part of your problem.**

Mistake 2:
NAPPING IN THE DAY

A daytime nap, on occasion, can be quite delicious. Many people grab 20 minutes on the train or the tube on the way to or from work. Others have a nap after lunch. On the odd occasion, napping is unlikely to have a detrimental effect, but if it becomes regular, it could start to affect your night-time sleep.

Some sleep specialists advise that a nap of under 20 minutes in the early part of the day is quite acceptable but on this programme it is not recommended. Daytime napping is playing with fire. Twenty minutes can easily turn into 30 minutes and then into an hour. And even a 20-minute nap will mean that when you finally get to bed at night, you may not be very sleepy, making it more difficult to drop off.

Additionally, some people find they can sleep anywhere *except* their own bed. This means that taking a nap on the bus or train reinforces their night-time insomnia. If you are one of these people, the most important thing you can do is to recreate the bed – sleep connection.

For all insomniacs, any napping weakens the connection between bed, night time, and sleep. So remember:

A nap in the day lessens your chances of sleeping at night.

Mistake 3:
LYING IN BED AWAKE

All insomniacs have had the experience of lying awake for hours, fidgeting and becoming more and more frustrated. This often happens when you have gone to bed before you are really sleepy. Insomniacs often make the mistake of going to bed 'because it's late' or 'because it's midnight', whether or not they feel remotely tired. Unsurprisingly, sleep does not come quickly.

Others may find it relatively easy to fall asleep but will wake up in the middle of the night and be unable to get back to sleep. As you lie there, desperate for sleep, you become tense and anxious. The tension you feel makes it impossible to relax and the bed seems to feel less and less comfortable as you toss and turn, trying to find a comfortable position. Your bed has now gone from being a sanctuary of peace and escape, to a place of misery and sleepless anxiety.

Remember:

**Every hour you lie awake in bed *weakens*
the association of bed and sleep.**

**Every hour you lie awake and frustrated *reinforces*
the association of bed with lying awake and being frustrated!**

Mistake 4:
LYING IN AT WEEKENDS

For many, the weekends are a great time to catch up on some missed sleep. Without the stress of having to get up for work, many people find that they tend to sleep much better on Friday and Saturday nights and may lie-in for hours in the morning, until 11 or noon. This may be the only decent sleep an insomniac gets all week and the joy of a delicious lie in is a temptation which few can resist. Others find that they do not sleep any better at the weekend than during the week, but even so, they usually get out of bed hours later on weekends compared with week days.

For many people, their only sleeping problem is so-called 'Sunday night insomnia' which means that the first day back to work on Monday is often marred by sleep deprivation. The reason for Sunday night insomnia is simply that, having overslept the previous two mornings, when you go to bed at your normal time on Sunday night, you simply are not tired. Thus it takes many hours to fall asleep.

It is also more than likely that much of the time lounging in bed was not spent sleeping, weakening the sleep – bed association.

Lie-ins are sleep thieves.

Mistake 5:
READING, USING YOUR LAPTOP, OR WATCHING TELEVISION IN BED

Many people turn to a book when they cannot sleep, or turn on the television in their bedroom. Others find the bed a comfortable place to work or study. Students, whose beds serve as both sofa and desk, often have problems sleeping. If your bed is currently serving as cinema, library and office, this is almost undoubtedly affecting your sleeping patterns.

When you do anything in bed, you are creating an association between your bed and that thing. This means that whenever you do anything in bed *other* than sleep you are, in effect, weakening your 'falling asleep response'. If you think about other associations you might have such as a biscuit with your coffee, tea in the afternoon or a snack in front of the TV, you will know how strong these feelings can be. Those of you who have tried to give up smoking will know that kicking the nicotine addiction is only part of the battle. Often much more difficult, is breaking all those strong associations of coffee – cigarette, beer – cigarette and after dinner – cigarette. If you are spending time lying in or on your bed to read, study, work or watch television, then you are weakening the bed – sleep association and creating a bed – being awake association. If your bed has become about everything *but* sleep, it is hardly surprising that you do not feel ready to drop off when you lie down at night.

Whatever you do in bed becomes associated with bed.

The Effects of Poor Sleep Habits

Before we go on, I need to say something about this first set of mistakes. They have been separated in order to draw attention to the importance of each. But all are concerned with a similar problem – *Poor sleep hygiene.* 'Sleep hygiene' is the term used for behaviour specifically associated with going to bed and sleeping. When one has '*poor* sleep hygiene' this alone is likely to lead to insomnia and for the majority of sufferers, is the root of their problem. While at university and also when self-employed, I was guilty of all five of the above mistakes. All of these things laid the perfect foundation for poor sleep to set in. Little wonder that I became an insomniac.

There are three main reasons that poor sleep hygiene can cause insomnia. The first two have already been covered in the previous pages. To recap, these are

1. *Anything* you do in bed other than sleep weakens the bed – sleep association and reinforces the bed – awake association.
2. Too much sleeping, either in the morning, at weekends or napping during the day, means you are not actually tired when you go to bed.

But there is a *third,* vital reason that poor sleep hygiene is so harmful, although you are unlikely to have heard of it.

The Stages of Sleep and Sleep Quality

Sleep specialists often claim that most people actually get a lot more sleep than they think. In tests, researchers claim that patients often report having no sleep whatsoever, while EEG results show that they have actually been asleep for six or seven hours. However, what is not made clear is that 'six or seven hours' refers to the *total* number of hours slept, with no mention of the *stages* in which this sleep occurred. In other words, no reference is made to the *quality* of the sleep had. Little comfort for those whose only problem is that their quality of sleep is poor – so that even a full night's sleep leaves them feeling unrefreshed.

The fact is that there are at least three distinct stages of sleep and in a normal night we spend varying amounts of time in each of them. A normal sleeper will only spend a few minutes in Stage 1 sleep before going into the deeper stages. But very often, patients in sleep clinics spend a much larger than normal proportion of the night in Stage 1.

In Stage 1 we may 'feel' we are still conscious even though we may dream quite readily. The rejuvenating effects of this type of sleep are minimal and without the deep and dreamless *Delta* sleep, one feels little if at all refreshed. It might be more accurate to describe Stage 1 as 'pre-sleep' or even 'non-sleep'. So, when you report 'I haven't slept for days', this is unlikely to be true. There are some nights when we actually get no sleep at all, but this cannot happen night after night. Like the sleep clinic patients, your sleep was probably so light that you mistook it for normal consciousness.

I, personally, have made the unpleasant discovery that while a night without any sleep is rare, it is quite possible to spend the *entire night* in Stage 1 – to go days, weeks even, having *only* this type of sleep. Insomniacs learn to *survive* on this tiny ration of poor sleep in the same way that a famine victim may survive for years in a state of near-starvation. But while it may be possible to survive *physically* on Stage 1 sleep, the emotional effect is devastating – the quality of life one has while getting only this type of sleep is wretched. In order to feel good in the morning you must spend a reasonable proportion of the night in the third stage – deep, *Delta* sleep. This is why you can spend 12, 13 hours in bed and feel worse than a night when you were only asleep for four hours. If those four hours included plenty of delta sleep, then they would have been far more beneficial than any number of Stage 1 hours.

Now, the link with this and sleep hygiene is this: when we spend too long in bed, we tend to spend a lot more time in Stage 1, and a lot less time in the refreshing delta sleep. Thus the *quality* of our sleep suffers. Eventually, the amount of Stage 1 sleep can approach 100% of the time spent asleep. Even today, there is a very clear direct link between the amount of purely Stage 1 sleep I get and the amount of time I spend in bed. If your problem is not with the amount but with the *quality* of your sleep you should pay special attention at this point. In a nutshell:

The *longer* you spend in bed the less chance you have of getting the *deep* sleep you need.

Shortening the time spent in bed increases the chance of getting the *deep* sleep you need.

The 'Psychological' Mistakes

These second set of mistakes are slightly different. They are not so concerned with sleep hygiene and bedroom habits, but rather with the ways that we create and reinforce negative *beliefs* about sleep. These may be more applicable to you long – term sufferers but even if your problem is a recent one, you may still find that parts of the following section apply to you. If you are a chronic long term insomniac it is likely that you have made several, if not all, of the following mistakes. While reading this section, bear in mind the following two negative facts of the mind which, in a nutshell, cover much of what is written below:

We tend to focus chronically on what we don't want
and
what we focus on gets bigger.
In other words,
the more attention you give to insomnia, the worse it becomes.

Mistake 6:
ASK YOUR DOCTOR FOR SLEEPING PILLS

Earlier in the book I described the many negative side-effects of sleeping medications. If you take a prescribed sleeping medication, you run the risk of developing addiction and many unpleasant physical and emotional problems. You may be more likely to crash your car, have accidents and your work and relationships may suffer. You may become depressed, anxious or even suicidal. Even the possibility of developing serious illness such as cancer and your overall mortality risk is increased.

Some research suggests that sleeping pills can help restore normal sleeping patterns if used for a short period of time, and perhaps they can in some cases. But are these few alleged successes really worth the countless horror stories of side-effects and addiction? The experiences of those who have come to me for help leads me to believe that the prescribing of sleeping pills for anyone is risky, at best. At worst, it is irresponsible verging on negligent. If you have, or know of a single person who has had a *fully* positive experience with sleeping pills, please email with the details.

Besides the more obvious negatives, sleeping pills can have an insidious yet devastating effect on your beliefs about sleep. So that far from curing insomnia, taking sleeping pills can actually *worsen* the problem. This is because when you take a pill for insomnia, you make two powerful and negative assumptions:

There is something wrong with me.

There is something external that can make me better.

This means that every night that you take a pill, you are reinforcing these two negative and erroneous beliefs. It's simple: when you swallow a pill, you say to yourself 'I can't sleep unaided' while at the same time investing that little tablet with the power to *make* you sleep. This means that any success in sleeping is attributed not to you, but to the pills. In basic terms, your belief is not in yourself, but in the medication. Thus your belief in your own ability to sleep is diminished. This negative reinforcement is one reason why, besides any physical addiction, sleeping medications are so powerfully psychologically addictive.

Many insomniacs prefer to self-medicate using alcohol. Because alcohol has a relaxing effect on the body it can help you to nod off. For some people it can also mask the effects of sleep deprivation, making an evening engagement tolerable when they have missed the previous night's sleep. But alcohol also dehydrates, depresses and can cause you to waken early with a full bladder, an adrenaline rush and a pounding heart as the chemicals leave your bloodstream. And of course there is almost always a degree of hangover when you wake after drinking alcohol which makes it unacceptable as a sleeping remedy.

There are also countless 'natural' remedies such as Valerian or over-the-counter medications such as Nytol. But just like prescribed medication, the only ones that have any effect will almost certainly leave you with some degree of drowsiness in the morning. And even 'natural' remedies hold a hidden danger: with all artificial sleep-inducing remedies, just as with prescription medication, you can come to trust and rely on the effect, making it impossible to rediscover and nurture your own natural ability to sleep unaided. Can you see how every time you take a prescribed sleeping pill, or self-medicate with 'natural' remedies or alcohol, you weaken your belief and so sabotage your natural sleeping capacity, pushing your recovery further and further away? When you go to bed, instead of trusting in your own ability to sleep naturally, you, in effect, hand over 'responsibility' to the drug. Your belief in yourself and consequently your own ability to sleep is diminished every time you take *any* artificial remedy. This is why artificial sleeping aids *cannot* ever help even a moderate insomnia problem. The message is simple: when it comes to sleep-onset or maintenance insomnia

Drugs don't work.

Mistake 7:
TRYING REALLY HARD TO FALL ASLEEP

Think about it: trying implies *effort* and unsuccessful effort implies frustration and tension, neither of which is conducive to falling asleep. Good sleepers don't 'try' to do anything and one thing is certain, if you try to fall asleep you will not succeed. This is because sleeping is not something you have to 'do'. Think back to a time when you did fall asleep easily. What did you do? The answer is that you didn't *do* anything. It might be more accurate to describe falling asleep as something you do *not* do.

Trying to fall asleep is a little like pushing really hard against a door which needs to be pulled – it's never going to open until you stop pushing.

The harder you try to fall asleep,
the harder it will be to do so.

Mistake 8:
OBSESSING ABOUT TIME

I do not advocate sleep diaries where every detail of one's sleeping and waking hours is recorded in term of hours and minutes. For people who are trying to stop obsessing about sleep, this is a terrible reinforcing behaviour. Clock-watching and box-ticking can create a horrible obsession with:

- time spent asleep
- time spent awake
- time spent before falling asleep
- time spent trying to fall asleep
- time spent waiting to feel sleepy after having got up after being unable to sleep.

Hence, one can feel tense and anxious in the morning, not because of sleep deprivation, but because of worries about the *number* of hours one has spent asleep. It actually doesn't much matter how *many* hours one spends asleep or waking because not all sleep is the same. All that matters is how one feels, and how well one functions in the daytime. We have all had perfectly happy and productive days in the past after only a few hours' sleep. Obsessing about the number of hours we *ought* to be sleeping makes the possibility of these carefree days more unlikely.

Clock-watching creates an unhealthy obsession with time.

Mistake 9:
TELLING PEOPLE ABOUT YOUR PROBLEM

It cannot be overemphasised how negative an effect talking about your problem can have. This certainly does not mean that you should sit on your problems, keep them hidden, and never speak about the fact that you are having difficulty sleeping. If it is really relevant to the conversation at the time, and you think that it might help your problem to mention it to a particular person, then do so. But when it becomes a real habit so that it becomes a topic of light conversation, something to mention as small talk or to someone you have just met at a party, something needs to change.

Perhaps you *never* talk to others about your problem. You may be one of those who 'bottles it up'. But be warned, all of the following points may still apply to you. It may just be that the only one you speak to about your problem is *yourself.* Monitor your inner monologue and look at the stories you tell yourself: how do you refer to yourself, what language do you use? Do the following points still apply, but only to your internal narrative?

Talking about your problem manifests in different ways in different people, but the following are particularly problematic.

Calling Yourself an Insomniac

Talking about your problem is particularly harmful if you are using your insomnia as a way of describing yourself – 'letting someone know a bit more about yourself'.

'I'm an insomniac.'

Can you see how destructive and negative and harmful this little phrase is? Labelling yourself with this term creates an identity, categorising you as one who is unable to sleep. By repeating this phrase you are describing yourself, your very *being,* in terms of a problem and so your insomnia becomes a fundamental part of who you are. People you know begin to ask 'how's your insomnia?' when they see you, reinforcing this identity. A negative feedback loop is thus created, with the message coming both from yourself, and from others, that you are ill, broken; that you are, *essentially,* an insomniac.

Simply giving a name to the problem goes a long way towards 'creating the monster'. By slapping a label on what is nothing more than a set of behaviours or events, we reify, or make real, a separate entity – *insomnia.* This term 'insomnia' implicitly suggests that an insomniac is suffering with a clearly defined medical condition, a disease one 'comes down with', one which requires medical attention, which must be 'cured' by the application of an external pill or remedy. *It is none of these things.*

Boasting

It's irritating, isn't it? Sometimes when you tell someone about your problem they claim, unjustifiably, *also* to be an insomniac when their problem is nothing like as bad as your own! 'Sometimes I lie awake for an hour!' they complain. An *hour*? What do they know? They know *nothing* about real insomnia! They don't know what it is to have it rule your life, to go days, months without proper sleep! You are going to tell them exactly what severe, chronic, long-term insomnia is like! After all, if anyone knows, *you* do!

Be really, really honest now: if someone tells you they have a sleeping problem do you feel compelled to boast about how much worse yours is?

I don't consider this to be boasting. I do tell people how bad the problem is, but it's only because I want people to know how serious the problem is. It is a large part of my life, a disability almost, and it is dishonest if I don't tell them the full extent of the problem.

Of course it doesn't feel like boasting. But exactly *why* is it so important to you that people know just how *bad* your problem is? Are you absolutely sure there is no satisfaction to be gained from seeing their horrified reactions, gaining their sympathy, and (you need to be really honest with yourself to admit to this one!) showing their problem to be insignificant compared with yours?

Exaggerating

Have you ever exaggerated your problem when telling others about it? Before claiming that you are not guilty, take the time to look within and be very honest with yourself. When you tell people your story do you tend to embellish it even a little when you tell them of the way it rules your life, or just how your problem is different?

Or do you exaggerate to *yourself*? Do your thoughts focus on those few really bad nights, playing them up in your mind, while ignoring the number of good nights of sleep you may have had? It's not that you have any intention of lying, or misleading anyone, it's just that a little exaggeration and boasting can be a very good way of making the seriousness of the situation apparent. The hitch here is that the boast eventually becomes reality, as the problem slowly begins to fit the exaggeration! At which point, a new *bigger* boast is needed – perhaps you now once went a *fortnight* without sleep. So be careful with exaggeration. Every time you exaggerate about how bad your sleeping is you create a new possibility for yourself. You give yourself something to live up to – a new goal to achieve, a new level of insomnia to work towards!

Some of you reading this book may only have had a problem for a few weeks, yet you may already be going around calling yourself 'an insomniac', and talking about your problem at every opportunity. The important message for *all* who have a problem sleeping is:

**The more you talk about, boast about,
exaggerate, and identify with your problem,
the worse it will become!**

No wonder sleep problems remain persistent. How are you ever going to change your beliefs about sleep if you are continually describing yourself as an insomniac and boasting in great detail about just how bad your problem is?

Some of you will have been suffering for decades and neither boast nor exaggerate. Indeed, many suffer in total silence and never talk to others about their secret problem. If this applies to you, do not be disheartened. If you don't do any of these things, great! Be happy that you have one fewer negative behaviour to change! But keep an eye and ear out for this tendency in yourself. It can be very insidious and you may need to be very vigilant to spot it, particularly if the one to whom you exaggerate is yourself. In short,

The story you tell about your sleep will come true.

Mistake 10:
RESEARCHING CURES IN BOOKS, MAGAZINES AND ONLINE

If you are a long-term insomniac, the chances are that you have tried countless cures and remedies in an attempt to overcome your problem. If you are new to insomnia it may not be immediately apparent what is wrong with researching things that might help, or with trying different remedies. But just how many sleep remedies have you tried? How many have failed to work? How much money have you spent on instant or 'miracle' cures? Do you find yourself buying any magazine or newspaper containing the word 'insomnia' or the phrase 'how to get a good night's sleep'? How many times have you inserted 'insomnia cure' into your internet search engine?

The internet is a massive, poorly regulated marketplace full of people attempting to make you part with your money. Sleep problems are big business with countless business people attempting to cash in on the desperation of the insomniac, and nowhere will you find more 'sleep cures' for sale than on the world wide web.

While we are living in a highly regulated world, where there are very strict limitations on what can be claimed in a television or magazine advertisement, the same cannot be said of the internet. Many internet businesses work by looking at what people are most desperate for, and by then making wild overblown promises that they can fulfil those desperate needs. 'Lose 60lbs in two weeks', 'make a £100k in a week', 'become irresistible to women', 'grow a larger penis', 'new wonder herb will make you sleep like a baby'. The claims we see on the internet, far from adhering to advertising guidelines, more closely resemble the outrageous claims of the Victorian side-show quacks and their wonder elixirs, 'guaranteed to cure all known ailments'. Incredibly, we actually fall for these scams, handing over our hard-earned cash on the promise of an unregulated website headline.

But why do intelligent people fall for these wild claims? The answer is simple: it's because we are *desperate*. The tragedy is that it is only the extreme level of desperation caused by insomnia which even makes it possible for these people to be in business.

But these outrageous claims and ineffective remedies do a lot worse than relieving you of £40 or £50. The damage is deeper and more subtle. Every time you send off for another ineffectual remedy you not only reinforce the idea that something is wrong with you. In addition, the suspicion begins to grow that your problem is special, chronic, *different*. When each of these nonsense cures fails to work, you imagine this must be because of the uniqueness or seriousness of your problem. It never crosses your mind that perhaps the 'cure' didn't work because the promises it made were nonsense in the first place. Peddlers of nonsense sleeping cures are doing more than taking people's money and not curing insomnia: they are actually harming people by making their insomnia worse! This is why the effect of useless sleep 'cures' is literally worse than nothing!

The Terrible Personal Laboratory

The belief that somewhere, somehow, there is one simple thing that we can take or do which will 'cure' us, combined with the sheer number of remedies out there means that our lives often become like a terrible personal laboratory where we become the subject of our own miserable, pointless experiments into sleeping problems. The more desperate we become the more combinations and concoctions we try. "Shall I take a pill, shall I take two Valerian and a glass of whisky? Shall I take half a Nytol and half a bottle of wine? Shall I wear earplugs? Shall I wear socks in bed? Shall I watch a film before bed? Shall I avoid an action/scary/film? Shall I exercise *then* have a hot bath with a glass of wine? Shall I have three large gins, two Nytol, a valerian tea, wear earplugs, socks and a hat, exercise just the right time before bed, try the new relaxation CD etc., etc., etc…?" Sound familiar? Just think about whether this sort of behaviour is actually good preparation for sleep? When bedtime arrives after such a mental tussle, are you likely to be in an ideal mental state for sleeping?

In desperation to be unconscious, some insomniacs will even take large, dangerous doses of medication combined with alcohol. Apart from possibly causing irreparable damage to the liver, these combinations are still often ineffective. The fact is we typically do such stupid things only when we are utterly desperate for sleep. But the sad truth is

People who are desperate for sleep do not sleep,
no matter what they do or take.

We have to shut down that terrible laboratory for good.

What are the special ineffective routines you do? In which ways do you obsess over tiny details of your life and pin hopes on little things which someone, somewhere in some article on insomnia suggested might help? Now think carefully before you answer the next question:

Have any of these things ever really helped?

The answer has to be a resounding 'no'! If these things were making a difference to your sleeping then you wouldn't be reading this book now. Some of these actions are more sensible than others, for example drinking strong espresso at 11pm may not be a good idea. But has watching scary films at night ever really caused insomnia? Has a herbal concoction ever cured a chronic insomniac? Have any of these things *ever* made a positive difference to a chronic insomniac? It's doubtful. But the *negative* effect that all these things have on a chronic insomniac is to increase the pressure, the obsessing, the wondering, the indecision, the not-knowing.

If you trawl the forum sites you will discover thousands of people looking for cures, or trying one sleeping pill after another, some of them suffering for 20 or 30 years! Why is it that none of them has ever found a cure, pill or remedy which has worked. The answer is simple: *they are looking in the wrong place.* The cure is not 'out there'! Chronic long-term insomnia is a problem which is largely caused by the thoughts you have and the beliefs you hold about the problem itself. It reacts to, and is worsened by, suggestion. No matter how long these poor people have suffered, until they are willing to look within, at themselves, at their thoughts and their behaviour, until they can square up to the suggestion that they are enabling their insomnia, until they can take an approach which is along the lines of this programme,

nothing will change for them, *ever.*

This is not like searching for a cure for dry skin, or mosquito bites, or arthritis, or cancer. Insomnia is a problem which assumes a life of its own. Feed it with fear and it grows. Constant researching and experimenting with cures is sustenance to the monster of insomnia. If you are a long-term insomniac you will probably have worked out that if only you could believe that you would sleep, if only you didn't fear insomnia, then you would be able to sleep. But how can you believe you are getting over your problem if you are still dedicating so much time to looking for a cure? Every time that you search for another cure or try the latest sleeping pill, you are saying to yourself 'I have a problem', 'I fear insomnia', 'I don't believe I can sleep'.

**If you are searching for miracle cures
you are looking in the wrong place.**

Mistake 11:
TESTING ONE RELAXATION METHOD AFTER ANOTHER

There are countless techniques and relaxation methods on the market that claim to help you sleep. These range from specific 'sleep entrainment' CDs to relaxation techniques and hypnosis. They are grouped together in one category because there is one simple reason why they so often do not work, particularly if your problem is well-established.

Most long-term insomniacs have gone through many, many relaxations CDs, mp3s and techniques.

That's me! I've tried them all; they don't work for me!

How do you know they don't work?

If you knew how many things I have tried you wouldn't ask that question!

But I *do* know! Why? – because I have probably tried them all myself. I was one of those people who had tried everything. I would give anything a go! People would say to me 'If I can't sleep I just watch my breath' or 'I tried the Fred Bloggs hypnosis CD and it put me to sleep in minutes' and my ears would prick up. If there was a new technique out there, I wanted to try it. I tried *everything*. Of course, I would always wait until a really high-pressure night to test the method 'properly'. There seemed no point in trying it on a night when I may have slept anyway because I would have been unable to tell whether the technique itself was effective. After all, what was the point if it wasn't going to work on the worst nights?

The odd thing was that whenever I tried a new relaxation method, or a technique designed to help me sleep, I found that it actually often seemed to make things worse! I would lie in bed, listening to my new hypnosis CD, or trying out my new relaxation method. I would start to relax deeply – on a physical level. But my mind would be alert, waiting to see what the effect was going to be of this unfamiliar bedtime companion. Eventually, I would start to become acutely aware of the fact that I was listening and acutely aware of the fact that I was relaxing. As you know, being acutely aware of anything is not particularly conducive to falling asleep. In fact, I started to become *awake*, wide awake. I was fully physically relaxed and about as far away from being asleep as it is possible to be! Failure! Another relaxation method was deemed ineffective, another CD was resold on Amazon marketplace and once again, something hadn't worked for me. I was still different, my problem was bigger, worse, more entrenched – I was just not like other people. My insomnia was quite unique, not like any of these 'everyday' insomniacs who could watch their breath for two minutes and fall asleep! What was different about me?

I could have kicked myself when I found out how simple the answer to this apparent problem turned out to be.

Why Relaxation Techniques Never Work for You

You probably are familiar with the phenomenon of people who live next to railway tracks or busy roads, who do not notice the noise of the trains or traffic? You will know exactly what I mean if you have ever moved into a noisy house or flat. For a week or two, you think you have made a terrible mistake, moving to a house where you can't sleep. You become miserable, being kept awake every night by the noisy trains or traffic passing by. But at some point, there comes a night where you sleep through the noise. Before long, you stop noticing the noise, and eventually you forget that you ever were disturbed in the first place.

I recently visited a friend who lives on a very busy road. I was astonished by the noise of the buses as they revved up waiting for the traffic lights to change outside the house and then as they pulled away. 'I don't know how you cope with the noise!' I remarked. 'Oh,' she replied, 'I don't even hear it.' We were then both reminded that less than a year ago when she had first moved in, she had complained bitterly about the constant noise of the buses in the street below. Now she had forgotten how it had once troubled her.

For some people, a very similar thing can happen with new techniques. After all, anything new and unfamiliar is likely to be interesting, stimulating or even threatening to your mind. Initially, the novelty will make you self-aware and anxious, and *this* is why it wakes you up. It is a form of defence mechanism which kicks in simply because something is unfamiliar. The first night that you try anything new is likely to be a disturbed night. However, in a week or so, you will have come to expect the recording or method when you go to bed. It will come to seem as normal as the presence of your pillow or the smell of the sheets. And so you begin to sleep, often much better than you had previously done.

If you 'test' the method on a high pressure night you have little chance of falling asleep. But once part of a normal bedtime routine, for some people the method can become a real comfort on those difficult nights.

So, it is the circumstances in which they are tried, and for how long, which are the the keys to making relaxation techniques work.

But why can some people be helped straight away by a technique or CD?

Look, we are all different. We aren't comparing like with like. The truth is that a lot of these people would probably have fallen asleep using any old technique or CD, by doing the head-to-toe relaxation, or watching the breath. You may just be one of those people for whom these things don't work straight away. You probably have an active, questioning mind which isn't going to trust something new and judge it to be safe and effective simply on the word of a complete stranger on a review site. You probably have a mind which likes to decide on things for itself. For people like you and me it is *only once* the technique has ceased to be unfamiliar that you can really judge its effectiveness. So whenever a person comes to me saying 'such and such relaxation method made me worse' my advice is always the same – 'try it again, every night for a fortnight'. The response is often overwhelming as many long term insomniacs find their sleep improving drastically from this advice alone. 'How could I be so *stupid,* ' one man wrote, 'not to realise this?'

If you are one of those for whom none of these things seems to work, you probably never tried anything more than once or twice before rejecting it, yes?

Yes, that's right. But that's because I was so desperate for sleep I thought it would be crazy to carry on using something that actually kept me awake.

I was one of those people who had tried everything – *once!* This was one of the greatest mistakes I made over the years. I constantly tried something once or twice and then rejected it. I wonder how many of those techniques might have worked, if only I had waited for the beneficial effects to show themselves. Who knows how many of these things might have worked like magic for *you*, if only you had stuck with them for a bit.

**Anything unfamiliar is likely to disturb sleep
for a period of time.**

Mistake 12:
VISITING INSOMNIA 'SUPPORT' SITES AND FORUMS

There is one sure way to turn a mild patch of sleeplessness into chronic insomnia – discover the online insomnia community.

I thought you said that they were lovely people?

And so they are. These are some of the kindest people I have ever come across and I am still in touch with many of them to this day. Your first insomnia forum will seem like a Godsend. There will be people here who really seem to care and who have the same problems. Finally, someone will understand what you are going through! Your stories will seem so similar and for the first time you may feel like someone is listening, that someone understands. You will find a worldwide community of well-meaning, caring individuals all with the same or a similar problem to your own, all talking, sharing, empathising, sympathising. There are insomniacs like you all over the world, millions of them, all suffering, none with a cure, none with an answer and all of them *constantly reinforcing each others' problems!*

If you are familiar with the sleep forums, you will know that when a forum member reads about a new 'cure' or research on a new approach, a new relaxation technique or a new herb to ingest, they will always check with the other forum members to get some feedback from someone who has already tried it. Hence they are full of messages from people asking: 'Anyone tried passionflower / NLP / acupuncture / magnetic therapy / colonic irrigation', etc. Sadly, anyone who asks a question like this is doomed to fail. Of course, they *want* to hear everyone say 'yes, passionflower tea cured my ten year insomnia problem overnight', but this *never* happens. Invariably, there will be a response from two or three from people who have tried (and failed) with those remedies. For the person who has posted the question there is nothing but disappointment as their hopes for the new remedy are dashed. 'If it doesn't work for them,' they imagine, 'it's bound not to work for me!'

It's essential to realise that insomnia forum sites and chat rooms are generally full of people looking for an answer to their problem, *not* with people offering a solution to a problem. Recovered insomniacs do not tend to hang around insomnia forums because they have usually worked out just how much this activity contributed to their problem. In the unlikely event that someone *had* cured a ten year insomnia problem with passionflower tea, the chances are that they wouldn't be available to answer any inquiries about it on an internet messageboard.

Worse than this, on internet forums you will also hear from people with real horror stories, much worse than your own. You may hear from people who have been searching for a cure for 30 years, people who have just relapsed after being 'cured', some claiming never, *ever* to have had a good night's sleep. Such stories can terrify a new insomniac.

I know what you mean. I hate to hear about people who have had insomnia for years and years. I worry that the same will happen to me.

Some insomniacs tend to identify with those with worse problems but never with those people who are helped by a simple remedy. For example, if a friend says to you: 'I couldn't sleep last year and I found that watching my breath really helped me' or 'a milky drink always works for me' you may not pay them any attention. On the contrary, you may find these people irritating! What do they know about insomnia? Watching the breath? Milky drinks? What nonsense! If they only knew what it was like to have *real* insomnia like *you* they would never say something so flippant!

Your situation may be no more similar to the person with the 30-year problem and who is addicted to sleeping pills than it is to the friend who cures a bad bout of sleeping with a simple 'watching the breath' trick. Yet we hear of a person with a situation which is worse than our own and we immediately begin identifying with them, even if in other ways their lives, personality and problems are nothing like our own. Then, before long this terrible self-fulfilling prophecy comes to be. Before long, their problems become our problems.

In general, established insomniacs tend to become irritated by success but identified with failure

One woman wrote to me reporting that she thought that certain types of insomnia were 'catching'. She explained to me that she had never in her life experienced a particular problem with having the cat on the bed. But she had read that pets should be kept out of the bedroom as their fidgeting can disturb sleep. Within no time, this problem had become her own. She was now shooing the cat out of the room and being disturbed by his crying at the door after 13 years of having him sleep peacefully on the end of her bed!

Insomniacs tend to absorb every little bit of negative information about sleep and make it their own.

How do you react when you hear a new piece of research or advice, announcing, for example, that drinking coffee after 12 noon can seriously affect your sleep? Do you take steps to stop drinking coffee after 12 *whether or not coffee ever really affected your sleep in the first place*? Insomniacs often have a long internal list of rules like this which may have nothing to do with their own situation. But because they are so obsessed with their own problem, they internalise someone else's rule about not drinking coffee. Yet another reason to panic, fret, worry and obsess about sleep rules.

Going on online chat-sites in order to help a sleep problem is a little like watching Crimewatch to lessen your fear of crime, or watching *Jaws* to get over your shark phobia. Insomnia forums are *not* support sites. Insomniacs cannot help you recover any more than heroin junkies can help you kick a drug addiction. They may be kind and sympathetic, but in general, they *cannot help.* It is true that there are a *few* kind souls who carry on posting about their successes, in order to help and inspire. But notice something – those recovered insomniacs never say 'I had a 15 year sleep problem and cured it with Valerian'; they inevitably tell a tale of slow self-realisation, a gradual change in belief and attitude and *always* a tale of good sleep hygiene.

Internet forums are not 'insomnia support sites'.
They are 'insomnia reinforcement sites'

Mistake 13:
REARRANGING YOUR LIFE AROUND YOUR INSOMNIA

It doesn't get any worse than this. There is perhaps no piece of behaviour which will accelerate the progress of your problem as much or hold it in place so firmly. If your insomnia problem has become so all-consuming that you are willing to compromise enjoyment of life rather than risk missing sleep, then you need to take action … now.

If you are a long-term insomniac, you are likely to be making many, many compromises to your life for the sake of sleep. If your problem is recent, check if you are already making small changes which impact upon the normal running of your life. Your particular behaviours are likely to be quite specific, which makes it difficult to identify them all. Such behaviours may include special routines; avoiding coffee even in the morning, avoiding *all* alcohol, avoiding scary films or spicy food at night, avoiding holidays or spending nights away from home, never staying out late, avoiding making plans, demanding special behaviours from your spouse or partner, or any other behaviour or special action (and this is the important bit) *intended only for the purposes of helping you sleep.* Many people even change their jobs in order to fit in with a sleeping problem. Becoming self-employed is common amongst insomniacs because of the mistaken impression that the greater freedom and flexibility of working hours will improve the chances of sleeping.

'Special Event' Insomnia

This problem is particularly pernicious if you have 'special event' insomnia like I had so chronically. It does not affect all insomniacs but I give it a special mention because it is one of the most stubborn forms of the problem. The fear of not sleeping before important events can seem impossible to overcome.

This was the last aspect of my problem to be eliminated, lingering long after I had otherwise recovered. And even though my sleep at this point was generally very good, I was still *terrified* of making plans. I never invited friends to dinner, or organised a night out or a party. I wouldn't even arrange a shopping trip or meeting someone for coffee or lunch. I stopped going on holiday and never, never stayed overnight at a friend's house. When invited to an event I would answer in the most disinterested way. 'I'm not sure what I'm doing yet', I would nonchalantly reply; 'can I let you know on the day?' A cast-iron plan was simply too frightening and by not committing myself to anything, I had a better chance of sleeping. To my close friends and family I even gave a set of rules: if you want to plan anything with me tell me about it on that morning. *Don't* tell me beforehand. Bless them; they stuck to my ridiculous rules. Any occasional breach of the rules would result in an angry response. I remember shouting at a friend for telling me about a future dinner party plan. 'Don't you know what you have *done*?' I shouted, 'You have condemned me to a sleepless night! How could you be so *thoughtless*?' What a nightmare I was living, and what a nightmare I was to live with!

I eventually found out that this was classic behaviour for someone with special event insomnia. I couldn't see it then, but every time I avoided making a plan, every time I feigned indifference to a social invitation, every time I demanded people follow my rules, and every time I reacted badly when they didn't, I was holding my problem firmly in place.

Some insomniacs simply refuse to attend social occasions or important events if they have not slept well and so begin missing out on all the good things in life, frequently cancelling or postponing engagements because they are too tired. Can you see how destructive this sort of behaviour is? Insomniacs will literally privilege the problem over their enjoyment of life. Are you beginning to compromise your normal life in order to avoid *any* danger of a sleepless night? In truth, there is no greater way to feed, grow and keep your insomnia monster healthy than by letting it dictate and affect your normal everyday activities.

When you start rearranging your life for insomnia, insomnia has become your life.

...5...

THE CURE

CHAPTER NINE

Introduction and Preparation

Introduction

Now that you have read and understood the ways in which we create and maintain insomnia, you may be starting to realise what sorts of things you are going to have to do in order to start your recovery. If so, the method is already working. But if not, do not despair. I am about to give you step-by-step instructions on how exactly to overcome your problem.

Just Make a Commitment

The Effortless Sleep Method insomnia programme consists of 12 *promises*, 12 commitments, *not* 12 cast-iron rules. Make these promises as part of an honest commitment to getting better and you become more than a rule-follower – you become responsible for creating a better life for yourself. Do not 'obey the rules' because someone is telling you what to do. Make the following promises because you understand the effect they will have on your sleep, and because you are fully committed to getting that sleep back to normal.

Making these promises should not be difficult. Stick to them with energy, with optimism, with dedication and feel *good* about it. Seen in this way, following the programme is not a hardship, it is an *empowerment. You* are taking control, *you* are taking responsibility, *you* are making the commitment to get over your problem.

Sleep Hygiene – The First Six Promises

Promises 1 – 6 of the Effortless Sleep Method are concerned with what experts call 'sleep hygiene'. This is a very simple non-drug solution which is effective in almost *all early cases of insomnia.* Sleep hygiene is really just a common-sense set of behavioural guidelines which help to restore normal sleeping patterns. If you have transient insomnia or have never tried sleep hygiene before, you may well be astonished by the speed at which these promises can make a difference. While simple, they are tremendously powerful and implementing good sleep hygiene at an early point will almost always stop a problem from becoming chronic.

If your problem is a recent occurrence or if you are not sure what sort of insomniac you are, you will still benefit from *all* of the advice contained in the Effortless Sleep Method. But, it may be best to begin by following the first six guidelines alone.

For most, sticking to the first six guidelines will be all that is needed to begin sleeping well again.

Those of you with a more serious or long-term problem must follow the entire programme – ***including*** the first six promises. Don't think you can skip the first six promises and move onto the more interesting bit! If you are a long-term chronic insomniac, you may well be very familiar with sleep hygiene rules. If this is the case, your response at this point might be 'been there, done that, didn't work'. But is this really true? I say this because most long-term insomniacs have, at some point, tried sleep hygiene rules, but a few sleepless nights here or there have resulted in their abandoning the whole idea. Is it actually that you believe your insomnia is just too severe to be helped by something so simple?

The fact is that when it came to curing myself, actually sticking to these guidelines had a *huge* effect on my sleeping habits, even after 15 years of chronic insomnia. These guidelines are *powerful* and it is amazing how much difference they can make. Sleep hygiene rules alone may not be enough to cure a chronic insomniac, but they do lay a very sturdy foundation of conditions conducive to sleep. These are the ideal circumstances for the other promises to work their magic.

So don't make things difficult for yourself: follow the sleep hygiene guidelines *even if you have tried them before* and give the rest of the programme a fighting chance to succeed. One thing is certain: you will have a very difficult job keeping the other promises if your sleep hygiene remains poor.

Whether you have suffered for years, or whether your problem is new, you *must* make the first six sleep hygiene guidelines a part of your life.

This programme is written, not just for the occasional, or new sufferer, but especially for long-term insomniacs. For many, negative beliefs and self-defeating contributory behaviours mean that, though essential, sleep hygiene *alone* may not be enough to overcome insomnia.

What's Missing from Traditional Sleep Hygiene? – The Second Six Promises

There are many books which offer solutions for sleeping problems. Almost all of these presuppose that insomnia is just about what goes on in the bedroom. The truth is that bad sleep habits often extend beyond the bedroom and into everyday life, and if you are a chronic insomniac, the essence of your recovery will be in learning to *believe* that you can sleep. The vital difference between this programme and others is that we address, not just the behaviours associated with 'going to bed', but also those specifically associated with, and which reinforce, negative thoughts and faulty

115

beliefs about sleep. Promises 6 – 12 are geared more towards those long-term sufferers, who are likely to have tried many remedies and techniques without success. These promises are more concerned with changing negative beliefs you may have about sleep.

The next section will explain how, in attending to negative behaviours, you will find the beliefs changing automatically and the problem falling away. The good news is that these behaviours are relatively easy to change.

Preparation – Make things easier on yourself

Before embarking on the programme, there are a few common-sense things you can do in preparation. These are not 'rules' or strict guidelines in themselves but are small lifestyle changes which many people find make sleep just that little bit easier.

Cut out stimulants before bed – After 15 years I still would hear people, including doctors, asking me if I had tried cutting down on my coffee intake. Sometimes my frustration would get the better of me, 'No!' I would say with feigned amazement, 'I had never thought that *coffee* might keep me up!'

In the unlikely event of your not knowing that coffee can keep you awake, and if you do drink several cups of coffee a day, or if you drink coffee or cola later in the day, be aware that this is likely to have a detrimental effect on your sleep. Similarly, if your favourite tipple is vodka and Red Bull, do not be surprised if you find it hard to sleep after a night out.

Coffee should be limited to one or two cups in the morning. If you are drinking more than this then there is a good chance that it will be affecting your sleep. And don't underestimate the effect of a strong cup of tea. Again, limit your tea intake and do not drink it in the evening. Cola drinks also contain a surprising amount of caffeine. So treat cola like coffee and avoid drinking it at night.

If you find yourself still feeling 'wired', even when it is time to go to bed, it may well be that you are very sensitive to caffeine. Bear in mind that caffeine sensitivity can develop at any point in your life, even if previously you have not found it particularly stimulating. Experiment with cutting down or eliminate it completely for a few weeks, even if you think it is not affecting you. Only then will you know for sure whether it is having an impact on your sleep. Giving up needn't be forever and you can always go back to drinking coffee and tea at a later date if you find that eliminating it makes no difference.

Get some exercise! – If you find yourself tired all day, but wide awake when it gets to bedtime, this is often because you have not had enough exercise. Going to bed at the end of a long tiring day is one of life's greatest free pleasures. If your muscles are tired, then getting into bed and resting can be quite delicious. Unfortunately, these days you are more likely to spend your working life hunched up in front of a computer screen all day or sitting at a desk. If you are very sedentary during the day, then even though you may be tired when you go to bed, your body will be tense and it will take you much longer to relax sufficiently to fall asleep.

Exercise also has an extraordinary effect on mood and can be very effective against depression. Join a gym or a class if you are so inclined, go for a brisk walk or jog, cycle or use a celebrity exercise DVD. It doesn't much matter as long as it makes you feel physically tired and a bit sweaty. You should aim to exercise at least three times a week. For insomniacs, a little every day is better than a hard workout once a week.

Sort out your environment – In the early days especially, do what you can to make your bed and bedroom as comfortable as possible. If your mattress is old and lumpy, change it. Buy some new 100% cotton bedding. And don't skimp on pillows and duvets. Buy the best quality you can afford. Many people spend more on a jacket or a pair of shoes that they wear for a few months, than they do on bedding that they use every night for years. If you are not allergic to feathers, a feather pillow and duvet are a worthwhile luxury. If you cannot afford such things then make sure your bedding is always freshly laundered. Buy some fabric conditioner with a nice smell, or add some starch to the wash to make the sheets crisp and inviting.

For many people, it is almost impossible to fall asleep if they are too cold and many find that simply being warmer in bed can eliminate a wintertime sleeping problem. Most people sleep best in a warm bed in a cool room. So turn the heating off and pile up the bed, or use an electric blanket. During the winter, wearing socks and putting a second duvet on the bed can make a huge difference. You can always kick them off if it gets too hot later. You need to be really warm and comfortable when you get into bed. If your insomnia is severe then the first few minutes in bed are crucial; if you have to spend this time 'warming up' you have a much poorer chance of falling asleep quickly.

If the weather in the summer makes it impossible to have a cool room, then experiment with a fan. Many people use a fan every night, even in winter, because apart from its cooling qualities, the 'white noise' it emits is very soothing and can be almost hypnotic.

In addition, most people sleep best in a very dark room. If the sun rises early where you live, use some blackout curtains to make sure the rising sun doesn't wake you before you are ready. You can also experiment with eye shades, but make sure these are loose and very comfortable – with Velcro fastenings. The elasticated ones found on aeroplanes are usually too tight and may end up disturbing you.

Chill out! – If you are a generally tense or anxious person then you will have a harder time than someone who tends naturally to be chilled. Set aside time for relaxation or meditation, even if it is only 15 minutes a day. You may be amazed by the effect that this can have on your life in general, and the more relaxed you are when you get to bed time, the greater your chances of sleeping. This is not the same as the bedtime relaxation techniques I speak of later in the book, but instead refers to how relaxed your 'background' state is, the state you are in when you come to bed. A *hot* bath or shower one hour before bed can be extremely helpful. Besides the obvious fact that a bath is enjoyable and relaxing, research has shown that as the body cools down, sleepiness sets in, reaching a peak one hour after the bath.

OK, are you ready? The essence of the Effortless Sleep Method is a set of 12 promises, 12 commitments to getting your life back. Some of these may sound familiar, but others will be quite unlike anything you have heard before, and are going to have an incredible effect on your sleep. All you need to do now is to keep to these promises and watch for the results!

CHAPTER TEN

The 12 Promises

Promise 1.
SPEND *LESS* TIME IN BED

Paradoxical but true! This one little promise is the simplest and yet the most powerful change any insomniac can make. Unbelievably, some 90% of you will be able to cure your problem with this promise alone! Spending *less* time in bed is undoubtedly the most effective treatment for all types of insomnia. So I cannot put this more strongly: if you are lying in late in the mornings or are going to bed earlier in order to catch up on sleep, then this must stop!

When you get into bed at night, it is vital that you are actually sleepy. While this may sound obvious, it is astonishing how often we get into bed not remotely tired and still are surprised when we have trouble dropping off. The longer you spend in bed, the less tired you will be the following night, and if you are not tired when you get into bed, you have very little chance of falling asleep. So, no matter how late it is, do *not* go to bed unless you are tired.

Next, you need to discover that number of hours of sleep that ensures you will be really tired when you go to bed. From now on, this must be the maximum time you spend in bed. You probably have a good idea of the amount of sleep which will ensure that you are really tired when you go to bed. But this is *not* sleep restriction therapy. You *also* need to feel good all day, function well, and not be overwhelmed by the desire for a nap in the afternoon. The ideal time seems to be between six and seven and a half hours for most people. But be honest about this, there is no point in saying 'I need nine hours' if you can really feel very good on six. What we are trying to do here is find the amount of sleep which will enable you to feel good all day, yet still means that when it comes to bedtime you are really tired and ready for sleep. This means that there is some resistance in the morning when the alarm goes off but once up and about, you feel fine for the rest of the day. Your mood should be good and you will be unlikely to nod off during a meeting or on the tube home. However, at bedtime you should be so ready to drop off that there is very little chance of your lying awake for more than a few minutes. If you find yourself waking up half an hour before the alarm goes off and dozing until it does, cut your time in bed back by half an hour and stop the extra dozing. The result will be that you still feel just as good all day, but will fall asleep much, much faster and will be less likely to wake in the night. Many people report that limiting their time in bed to just the right number of hours has allowed them to sleep through the night for the first time in their lives.

You will need to experiment to find your ideal time to spend in bed. A good rule is to start with the amount which seems right to you, minus half an hour.

> If you don't see an improvement in your sleep within a week, cut the time spent in bed by half an hour.

> If you see an improvement in the time taken to fall asleep, but find yourself unbearably sleepy during the day, increase the time by half an hour.

It is important not to be too rigid about these 'rules'. The more regimented a sleeping plan, the more likely it is to become a crutch. Remember, this method does not work by making you *desperate* for sleep, like sleep restriction therapy. The method works in many subtle ways to change the way you think and act regarding sleep. Most importantly, the changes you make will improve your attitude and beliefs about your problem, and these beliefs are not created or destroyed by one night's sleep or lack thereof. This means that there is much greater leeway for the *occasional* mistake.

As long as you don't flagrantly abuse and disregard the guidelines, the odd *accidental* oversleep will not affect the effectiveness of the method. But be warned, if sneaky lie-ins, excused as accidents, become commonplace, you effectively sabotage your recovery. The point is to be *tired and sleepy* when you go to bed. If you are not, the insomnia may return.

**90% of all insomniacs can be cured
by simply spending less time in bed.**

Promise 2
NO NAPS

From now on, avoid napping in the day at all costs. If napping in the day is the only decent sleep you get, it will undoubtedly be at the expense of a proper full night's sleep. Sacrifice the nap, not the night.

You should never *plan* to get a nap on the train, but don't get into a panic if you do! Don't beat yourself up over it. Instead, use it as a reason to give yourself a little pep-talk to bolster your confidence. 'Look how well I slept on the train!' tell yourself, 'I *never* used to be able to sleep like that!', 'I must be getting better', 'I should be able to sleep like that at home too!'

But *don't* let the naps become the norm or they will begin to affect your chances of sleeping at night. If you consistently find it impossible to stay awake on the train or bus, lengthen your time in bed by half an hour and see if this helps.

Sacrifice the nap for the sake of a full night's sleep

Promise 3.

GET UP AND DO SOMETHING WHEN YOU CAN'T SLEEP

So, what do you do when sleep just doesn't come? Well, the one thing you shouldn't do is to continue to lie there, not sleeping. If you can't sleep you should get out of bed. There are two different reasons for this. Firstly, like the other sleep hygiene rules, every minute that you lie in bed, wide awake, reinforces the connection between bed and anxiety, and weakens the connection between bed and sleep. But secondly, the fact is, you are more likely to fall asleep very shortly after getting into bed, when the 'sleepy feeling' appears. If you lie awake once that feeling has come and gone, it can take a very long time lying there for it to return. In some cases it simply will *not* return until you get up and change your surroundings.

The advice found in almost every insomnia book or set of guidelines is that if you are not asleep within 20, or in some cases, 15 minutes, you should get out of bed and do something boring until you feel ready to fall asleep. This is an effective rule, but in most cases, the rule does not need to be so strict. I don't now, and never did, even as a child, fall asleep within 20 minutes. Perhaps this is another example of a rule being written by someone who has never missed a night's sleep in their lives. If you have lain comfortably in bed for 20 minutes but still feel drowsy and sleepy there is often a very good chance that you will still fall asleep quite soon.

So, don't be too concerned with the actual number of minutes that you have lain awake. The Effortless Sleep Method rule is rather: get up and do something 'when you can't sleep'.

So what exactly does this mean? Well, if you are like most insomniacs then a bad night goes something like this – You close your eyes and begin to become sleepy and drowsy and less aware of your surroundings, just like any normal sleeper. You may be on the verge of sleep when, suddenly, you awake with a jolt. Or, you may just slowly become aware of the fact that you have been in bed for some time but aren't asleep. At this point you probably start to become more awake and the 'sleepy feeling' begins to diminish. You are waking up, not getting sleepier. When it is unmistakeable to you that this is happening, *this* is the time to get out of bed. This may be after five minutes or an hour, it doesn't much matter.

But what to do when you do get up? Many experts advise you to do something boring when you get up, like reading the phone book. You can do something boring if it helps; any change in focus is usually enough, whether it's having a hot bath or shower, doing some housework or taking the dog out for a walk. But what is *very* important is that you have worked out what you will do should you wake up *before* you lie down to sleep. This will make it much easier to drag yourself out of the warmth and comfort of your bed. Have a jigsaw puzzle ready on the table, have in mind to clean the skirting boards, or a particular bit of studying to do. Many great writers were night owls, writing some of their best work in the small hours when the rest of the world was asleep. So perhaps have a piece of creative writing in mind. As long as the activity is not extremely stimulating, such as vigorous activity which can make it difficult to fall asleep quickly afterwards, it doesn't much matter what it is. Most people complain of not having enough time in the day to get everything done. If you are an insomniac, don't ever let this be the case. Fill those night-time waking hours with meaningful activity and feel the satisfaction at having got so much more done. Going to bed with a plan for what you will do if you need to get up can also lessen your anxieties because the pressure to sleep is less: if you sleep – great! If you don't – you'll do the ironing. Simple as that. Some examples of ideal things to do are:

- Jigsaws
- Cleaning out the fridge

- Cleaning out kitchen cupboards
- Having a hot bath or shower
- Doing a crossword or Sudoku
- Doing one of the relaxation techniques in the next chapter

If you really cannot summon the willpower to get out of bed and undertake some activity in the middle of the night then there is a compromise move you can try, although it is probably not a good idea if you are elderly or have circulation problems. Instead of carrying out an activity, get out of bed and lie on the cold hard floor in your bedroom or in another room. Do not snuggle up with a blanket. The idea is *not* to be comfortable enough to fall asleep. Lie there for *at least* 20 minutes and then go back to bed. Try counting to 60 on each finger, twice. This is particularly effective if you have an electric blanket to return to when your bed will seem so warm and inviting. Sleep will be much easier to find.

The other important thing about any night-time activity is that whatever you decide to do, it should be a job which can be finished in between 30 minutes to an hour. If you get up and just 'do some cleaning' with no thought of what you might do, you may find yourself idly dusting until it feels like about 30 minutes has gone by. The idea is that your focus is taken away from clock-watching, away from the fact that you are not asleep. It could have a negative effect if you are constantly focussed on the fact that you are doing an 'insomnia activity'. So don't get up and 'do some cleaning', get up and clean out the fridge or dust every skirting board in the house. In this way, your focus is on the activity, not on whether it has been 30 minutes since you got up. It needs to be just long enough so that when you get back into bed, it feels relaxing and fresh, and that you can start the 'falling asleep' process all over again. Then the sleepy feeling will come over you anew, and you will have a much better chance of falling asleep this time.

Do not decide to break this promise just because it doesn't work the first few times you try it. In the early days, this promise is likely to interfere with your sleep and you may have a few sleepless nights because of it. But you must persevere. This guideline is designed to break a negative association; it is not an insomnia cure in itself.

If you are in bed you should be asleep.
If not, get up.

Promise 4.
GET UP AT THE SAME TIME *EVERY* DAY

This simple and seemingly unimportant little promise can have the most incredible effect on sleeping patterns. Without a regular getting up time, all the other sleep rules have much less chance of working. And before long, getting up at the same time at weekends will no longer bother you one jot.

When this promise is combined with promise 1, 'spend less time in bed', the two create a powerful foundation for all other sleep promises. It is these two which lay the most important condition for sleep to occur – that you are actually tired when you get into bed! Without these, you might as well forget the rest of the programme.

Once you have decided how long you need in bed, work out the time at which you will be able to get up, not just during the week but at the weekend too. If you need seven hours to feel good all day, yet are still sleepy at bedtime, and you must get up at 7.30 on weekdays, then you must also get up at 7.30 on weekends. There will be no more lying in at weekends, so try not to have too many late nights, at least in the early days.

This will seem harsh to you if the weekends are the only time you currently get any decent sleep, but when you begin to notice the effect this has on your sleeping patterns, it will no longer be a hardship. Remember, insomnia often sets in during self-employment, university, illness or unemployment – in other words, at a period in one's life when there is no necessary compulsion to get out of bed at the same time every day.

Besides the fact that you are actually tired when you lay down to sleep, the psychological effect of knowing that you didn't sleep late in bed in the morning will provide comfort and increase your motivation to stick to the programme. It won't be long before you will begin to enjoy getting up at a good hour on the weekends. You will have more of the weekend to enjoy and will get a really positive boost from knowing that there is every chance that you will sleep well again the next night.

Good sleep loves routine.
Keep to yours and good sleep will become a habit.

Promise 5.

DO NOTHING IN BED BUT SLEEP OR MAKE LOVE

The main reason for all sleep hygiene rules is to create such a strong connection between bed and sleep that just the act of getting into bed and lying down triggers the falling asleep process. It is true that for many normal sleepers, reading or watching television in bed may not cause a problem. But at least in the early days, avoid doing anything in bed other than sleeping or making love. From now on these are the only two activities which are to take place in your bed.

So why is sex OK? If you really wanted to be strict about the rules, you could make sure that sex took place in another room, and never in your bed. However, unlike other activities, sex is unique in that it is a relaxing, de-stressing activity which often happens in bed, just before falling asleep. When it is over, it is time to sleep. Thus it already has an inbuilt association with sleep. Sex also releases endorphins, giving you a happy, warm and glowing feeling when you lie down to sleep. And best of all, unlike reading or watching television, which can go on indefinitely, sex has a finite duration. It is for all these reasons that many people find sex can almost instantly send them to sleep (and hence why women often complain that 'he just rolls over and falls asleep'!) This is why you must implement a 'sleep and sex only' rule.

The idea is to create an association of bed – sleep which is so strong, it will overcome all the stresses and fears you may have which are preventing you from sleeping. That association will eventually become so strong that you will be starting to nod off almost before you put your head on the pillow. That sleepy feeling will come over you at the very *thought* of your soft, warm, comfortable bed. Your bed means sleep – simple as that.

When in the throes of severe insomnia, your bed can become a place of misery and fear. But because of the combined sleep hygiene rules, the time in that bed will be rationed to only those hours when you are asleep or falling asleep. The result is that going to bed will become a treat you can look forward to all evening. Before long, you won't be able to wait to get into your delicious bed, between the crisp, white sheets, put your head on your soft downy pillow and pull up your warm, snugly duvet. Your bed will go from being a place of tension and misery to a sanctuary of peace, your own special little place in which you can curl up at the end of the day.

Bed = sleep or sex

Promise 6.
REDUCE OR ELIMINATE THE PILLS

IMPORTANT: you *must* get proper medical advice before starting any drug withdrawal programme. If you currently take a sleeping pill every night, particularly if it is a benzodiazepine or a Z-drug then you **must** speak to your doctor first about giving it up. I may know about the psychology of insomnia but I have little professional or personal knowledge about the chemical and physical side-effects of withdrawing from your particular drug. **Don't take a risk, get advice.**

The aim of this programme is to rediscover and rekindle your own, natural ability to sleep unaided and the taking of sleeping pills is in direct opposition to this approach. So for this programme to have a chance of working, it is essential that you are actively taking steps to reduce or stop taking medication in order to avoid sending contradictory and confusing messages to your unconscious.

If you take a prescribed sleeping medication, make an appointment to speak to your doctor about reducing your dosage. Resist any encouragement to trying a different, or a 'new' kind of pill unless it is prescribed specifically as part of your withdrawal programme. There is, at present, no new type of pill which works in any substantially different way to your current medication. Until a drug is developed which somehow induces real, natural sleep rather than simply doping the patient into a drugged stupor, this will remain true. Similarly, if you are regularly self-medicating using alcohol, you will need to take steps to reduce your consumption with a view to giving up altogether. This does not mean that you can never again touch a drop of alcohol. The rule is that you do not use alcohol *in order to help you sleep.* This is essential in order to instil the ability to attain natural, delicious sleep, without hangover or come-down, which can occur after drinking alcohol or taking medication. If you only occasionally take a sleeping pill, or regularly take over-the-counter medications such as Nytol or Sominex, you can stop taking them immediately.

As your recovery progresses, you will quickly reap the benefits of this promise. But to start with, there is a good chance that your insomnia will worsen for a time. This is the well-documented 'rebound insomnia', which is a common side-effect of giving up sleeping medication. If this happens to you, you have my every sympathy, but do your best to see it through. Sooner or later, you will begin to sleep again. Your first night's sleep with reduced medication will be a triumph, a success, *proof* that you are on the road to recovery. Every night that you sleep with reduced medication, or without medication at all, you send a powerful message to your brain; *I am getting better!* So, at some point, when you are no longer taking a nightly sleeping pill, you will need to make a commitment: *I will never again rely on sleep medication.* Making a commitment like this is a very empowering act. It implies that your insomnia is no longer running the show. *You* are back in control, of your insomnia and of your life.

At the end of the day, it is really up to you whether you decide to give up your medication or not. This is not a decision which should be taken lightly and must be made with the collaboration of your doctor. However, *if* you want to follow the Effortless Sleep Method then you will need to take steps towards giving up the pills. If you are not willing at least to take steps towards reducing the dosage of the pills that you currently take, the programme is not for you.

This method will give you something far more trustworthy and powerful than any pill. The Effortless Sleep Method aims to strengthen your belief in yourself, rediscovering your own inborn ability to sleep. In my opinion, anything less is unacceptable. Being able to sleep naturally and unaided, waking refreshed in the morning is the dream of every insomniac. *This* is true recovery from insomnia. *This* is what the Effortless Sleep Method can give you.

**Every night you sleep with reduced medication
is a step on the road to recovery.**

Promise 7.
STOP CLOCK-WATCHING

From now on, pay no attention to the number of hours of sleep you get. Work out how many hours you need, set your getting up time and from then on, *forget about time.* Do not have a clock in your room which can easily be seen. Turn the clock away from you or put it on the other side of the room. If you use a mobile phone to wake you, turn it off and do not look at it in the time between lying down and when it goes off in the morning. From now on, you should have *no idea* how many hours you slept last night, or how long it took you to fall asleep, or how early you woke in the morning. All that matters is how well you feel during the day.

It's *quality* of sleep, not quantity, that counts.

Promise 8.

REPLACE NEGATIVE SLEEP TALK WITH POSITIVE STATEMENTS

This promise is perhaps the most powerful aspect of the whole programme. From now on, you must make the following commitment:

No negative sleep-talk.

Telling people about your insomnia can have a devastating effect on your problem. However, its opposite – talking positively about yourself – can have a tremendously beneficial effect. From now on, avoid saying 'I'm a terrible sleeper', 'I'm an insomniac', 'I'm so tired today', 'I wish I had slept last night', and instead begin to look for positive things to say about your sleep. It will sound like a lie to begin with so start small, congratulating yourself for small wins – 'I slept pretty well last night'. The next time you have a good night's sleep, or even a *better* night's sleep, celebrate it, revel in it, telling yourself that you seem to be getting better. Make a point of telling someone 'I had *such* a good sleep last night', I slept like a *log* last night' or even 'I could have slept in for *hours* this morning'. See how it feels to say this. Isn't it empowering? It makes you feel like one of the 'normal' people, that you have joined the rest of the world. Can you see what has happened when you do this? You have actually become one of the people who boasts about how *good* their sleep is!

Use Affirmations

Affirmations have been given a very bad press in recent times, perhaps because unscrupulous salespeople have often claimed that one can achieve all manner of unlikely things with them, from attracting the mate of your dreams to becoming an Olympic athlete. But when it comes to sleep, we can be absolutely sure that positive affirmations *do* work simply because of the incredible success of *negative* affirmations.

The truth is, we are all constantly using affirmations that successfully reinforce our beliefs. The unfortunate truth is that these are usually *negative*. Telling yourself and others how bad your insomnia is is actually just a type of affirmation. Every time you think or say 'nothing works for me' or 'I'm a terrible sleeper' you reinforce the already strong belief that you are a terrible sleeper and that nothing works for you.

But if negative affirmations like this work so well, this must also be true for positive statements. For example, if you constantly tell yourself that you are getting better, you reinforce the belief that you are indeed, getting better. Positive affirmations are *very* powerful and if used properly will really speed up your belief change regarding insomnia. You have undoubtedly been using negative affirmations for years, so you should have no resistance to making this promise.

Imagine that instead of telling your friends, family and everyone you have met over the years about your bad nights of sleep, you instead had only boasted about the good nights. Can you see the effect that this would have had? Are you starting to have an inkling of the way you have created your own problem, your own reality? You know those people who hear of your sleep problem and respond by saying 'Oh, I can fall asleep anywhere', 'I'm a brilliant sleeper', 'I sleep so deeply that I need two alarm clocks to wake me'? How they annoy us ... and how we envy them! Well, the truth is, *you are only a short way from becoming one of them!*

Write it Down

Apart from stopping negative private and public self-talk, you can make your affirmations a little more structured and formal. Buy a nice A4 lined pad and use a pen which is comfortable to use. A fountain pen or gel pen is ideal. Now, every day you will write out, in neat handwriting one of the following affirmations.

I am a brilliant sleeper.
I am amazed at how well I sleep now.
I can sleep anywhere, any time.
I really enjoy going to sleep at night.
I love sleeping.
I can sleep better than anyone I know.

If you want to make up your own affirmation script this is fine, but please do bear the following in mind: Psychologists know that the unconscious mind responds only to positive *statements*. So avoid using words like 'not', 'never', 'haven't, and words like 'problem', 'insomnia' and 'bad'. Affirmations should always be written in the present tense and should be *statements* communicating situations, facts, or possible states of affairs, *not* wishes, hopes or worries. So the following affirmation would be fine

I really am getting better.

But these would *not* be helpful.

I hope I won't have this sleep problem for much longer.
I really want to get over my insomnia.
I really hope I can sleep tonight.

Fill the whole page with one repeated affirmation, and as you write, think about the meaning of the words. Don't rush. If you treat it as a chore to be finished as soon as possible then it will not be as effective. Write with care and feeling. You can also say the words as you write. Think about what the words mean and allow thoughts and pictures to come into your head which fit them. I like to fill the line and write the sentences directly under each other so that the finished sheet looks something like this

I can sleep SO well, better than anyone I know.
I can sleep SO well, better than anyone I know.
I can sleep SO well, better than anyone I know.
I can sleep SO well, better than anyone I know.
I can sleep SO well, better than anyone I know.
I can sleep SO well, better than anyone I know.
I can sleep SO well, better than anyone I know.
I can sleep SO well, better than anyone I know.
I can sleep SO well, better than anyone I know.
I can sleep SO well, better than anyone I know.
I can sleep SO well, better than anyone I know.
I can sleep SO well, better than anyone I know.
I can sleep SO well, better than anyone I know.
I can sleep SO well, better than anyone I know.
I can sleep SO well, better than anyone I know.
I can sleep SO well, better than anyone I know.
I can sleep SO well, better than anyone I know.

When the page is full it looks neat and attractive, like a work of art, a poem. It will give you a pleasing psychological boost to see the finished page.

People with positive ideas about their ability to sleep do not find ways in which to be different, make their problem unique, or boast about their problem and how bad it is, and from now on, neither will you. People with positive ideas about their ability to sleep boast about how well they can sleep – 'I can sleep through any alarm' and even exaggerate about how well they can sleep - "I could sleep on the pavement of Piccadilly Circus! Neither the positive nor the negative exaggeration is a truer reflection of reality. So from now on, just *choose* the exaggeration that makes you feel better! To start with, this will all seem silly, like a big lie. But I promise you, before very long, these words will start to ring true. One day, instead of thinking 'what a load of rubbish, I'm not a good sleeper no matter how many times I write this', you will start to entertain the thought 'maybe I really am a good sleeper now'. When this happens, it will be a real turning point in your recovery. From then on you will be amazed at how quick and powerful an effect such continued affirmations can have on your beliefs.

**Start writing your own story,
and it will come true.**

Promise 9.
LET GO OF THE SEARCH FOR AN INSTANT MIRACLE CURE

If you are a long-term insomniac, this might just be the hardest, and the most important promise of all. Let go of your search and you let go of one of the main culprits which is keeping you wedded to your problem. If you are looking for an external cure then you are looking in the wrong place, simple as that. The way to cure insomnia is to look no further than your own thoughts and behaviour. Remember, it is not just your lack of sleep that is the problem; it is your beliefs, your thoughts and your contributing behaviours that hold this problem firmly in place, and searching for a cure is one of those contributing behaviours!

You must stop searching for cures in magazines and in books. Throw out all remedies and potions, tapes and CDs. Cancel your subscription to any insomnia newsletters. Tell any online forum friends that you will be out of circulation for a while. In your mind you must accept that the search for an external cure is over. In order to do this, there is one fact that you are going to have to accept right from the start:

This is not going to be cured overnight.

But I want it now! I need it now – I just don't have enough self-belief to even start thinking positively until I get a few good nights' sleep. Recovery has to be quick or I will simply give up.

Your recovery may well be quick. You may well start sleeping better from tonight. But you must allow your recovery to take as long as it needs to. If you demand that a cure be instant then you are likely to view a single missed night as failure or proof that the method doesn't work. In this case you will be doomed to fail. I can say with absolute certainty that you will never find a pill, potion, technique, method or cure which will instantly and overnight cure your insomnia. I can say categorically that there *is* no external, *instant* miracle panacea for insomnia.

Does this thought still worry you? If so, then consider this: what if, hypothetically, it took a *year* to beat this problem? A whole year! Does this strike you as totally unacceptable? Think about it for a moment. What if it took a *whole year* for you to be insomnia free…?

… then in a year's time you would be ***insomnia-free.***

And now consider this: what if you refuse to give up the idea that somewhere there exists a medication or external remedy that will cure you? What if instead, you continue to research cures for a whole year …

… then in a year's time you will be ***in the same position you are in now.***

So the choice is yours: at some point in the future, be it a week, a month or a year, you can be sleeping naturally, effortlessly, like a baby. Or, you can continue to search aimlessly *and in the wrong place* for the mythical panacea for insomnia. In which case you can be certain of this: in one year you will be exactly where you are now. Take your pick. The fact is: *you are now on the road to recovery.* If this is true, what does it matter how long that road is?

You are on a programme that works, and as long as you stick to it, you *will* get better. Soon, you will know with great certainty that this is true. One morning you will wake up surprised that you have slept so well. And the realisation that you are genuinely, indisputably regaining your natural ability to sleep is worth all the money you could ever spend on nonsense cures.

All you need to cure yourself is within you.

Promise 10.
DISCOVER A RELAXATION TECHNIQUE THAT WORKS FOR YOU

If your busy, active mind is stopping you from sleeping, it is important to have some way of switching off the obsessive thinking and worrying which can keep you awake. In the next chapter you will find 'relaxation techniques' designed for all manner of people.

As I have explained, for many people, especially long-term insomniacs, a new technique will only work once it has become established as a part of their bedtime routine. So pick a relaxation technique that appeals to you and commit to using it every night until it ceases to feel new. Start using it on a low-stress night, not on a night where there is great pressure on you to sleep. Continue to use it every night until it begins to feel normal and familiar, even if to start with it seems to make your sleeping a bit worse.

It is recommended that you use either the Effortless Sleep Tools, or use one of the techniques laid out in this book. You may need to try a few to find one that suits you as not all will have the same effect on each person. For example, I find progressive body relaxation useless; others swear by it. But in each case, do not reject something until you have used it nightly for *at least* a fortnight. In this way, when a high-pressure night comes along, it will be so familiar that it will act as a comfort, rather than a disturbance.

This may seem to contradict all I have said about crutches, and the way we can come to depend on them. But remember, there is nothing *intrinsically* harmful about using a crutch, as long as it is harmless, is reliable, and most importantly, that it is used alongside attention to faulty beliefs. Ultimately speaking, the only crutch

143

worth having is belief in your own ability to sleep. But for some, this is too big a jump to make. And for those, a relaxation CD or technique is a fine intermediate stage. *This* is why it is recommended that you find a relaxation method that works for you. If at some point you feel the technique has become a crutch, then it is up to you when and if to eliminate it. If you do decide to eliminate it, the very next promise will be essential. For now you simply need to remember:

**Relaxation techniques and recordings
will usually only work once they have become familiar.**

Promise 11.

DECIDE ON YOUR OWN SAFETY THOUGHT

The Best Ever 'Crutch'

The problem with crutches is that eventually they are liable to let you down. Because they are external things, they really have nothing intrinsic to do with helping you sleep. What they give you is a safety net, something to believe in, something to trust when you feel anxious.

The terrible personal laboratory is now permanently closed for business. In its place we need to position your own personal safety net, your 'safe thought' which calms and soothes you when you are worried about whether you will sleep. When the panic comes over you and thoughts of not sleeping fill your head, you simply need to remind yourself of your safety thought.

Can you remember a night, or a stretch of nights when you slept really well? Can you remember a time when you didn't expect to sleep and yet still did? Can you remember a night when even though you were anxious about sleep, you still somehow managed to drop off? It may have been quite recent. Try to find a comforting and encouraging *fact* about your sleep – not wishful thinking, a *fact.* Have you had even *one* good night's sleep recently? Pick whatever positive fact you feel would be most likely to give you hope during the stress of the day and in the dark lonely nights in bed. Some examples are:

1. You may find that sometimes you will sleep even though you go to bed in an anxious state. The safety thought might be: *I slept through anxiety like this before and I can do it again.*

2. You may find that you have a 'high-pressure' night – in a hotel or strange bed or before a vital event and still manage to sleep like a baby. The safety thought would be: *I slept before on a high-pressure night so I can do it again.*

3. You may find that you apparently do not sleep at all, or at least very badly, and yet enjoy the following day so much you forget that you had even missed a night's sleep. The safety thought would be: *It really doesn't matter whether I sleep or not.*

Now, it is very likely that at some point since your insomnia started, at least one, if not all of these things have happened to you. But for some reason, these occasions in the past have been pushed to the background, covered up and ignored. From now on, they will take centre stage. These occasions when you slept in non-ideal circumstance *prove* to you that you are normal. Now your safety thought can be:

I can sleep no matter what.

For me the first safety thought was the knowledge that I *had* occasionally slept really well for a stretch of three to four nights. I would tell myself: *tonight might be the beginning of a good stretch.* This gave me a sense of peace so strong that even on the worst nights of the early days of my cure it was often enough to let me fall asleep.

My safety thought changed as I recovered, and I became more free and adventurous with my plans. Eventually, towards the end of my recovery, it became the thought that even before *really* exciting things still *occasionally had slept.* I would remember a time when I had slept on a very high-pressure night, perhaps before a wedding. I would then remind myself of this fact during the day, and as I lay in bed, basking in its safety – 'I did it once, I can do it again', 'I *can* sleep before fun events'.

If you find it hard to find a positive fact about your sleep, make your safety thought your promise or commitment to the behavioural changes you are making. Your safety thought could simply be: *I have stuck to the programme, I am getting better!* Unlike the affirmations previously mentioned, your safety thought must be a *fact.* You can lie down at night knowing that it is a *fact* that you got up at a good hour, that you didn't have a nap, that you didn't moan about your insomnia today. You have stuck to a plan which works and, therefore, done *all* you can to give yourself the best chance of sleeping. There is nothing more to decide, nothing to wonder about, nothing more to do! Feel *good* about that fact! Relax into your safety thought and let go into the night.

And the wonderful thing about this safety net is that there are no negative side-effects! However, there are a myriad of positive side-effects!

Remember the two important principles mentioned above: we tend to focus on what we don't want, and what we focus on tends to get bigger. Of course, the flip side of this is that if we focus on what we *do* want, that gets bigger also. And that is how the positive safety net becomes stronger every time you lie into it. So, decide on your particular safety thought for the night, hold onto the thought, bask in it, relax into it. And then let go.

Your safety thought will support you as you fall.

Promise 12.

PUT YOUR LIFE
BEFORE YOUR INSOMNIA

Do you avoid situations which might affect your sleep such as fun events, camping trips or staying overnight with friends? Do you leave parties early so you can get to bed at a good hour? Do you refuse to stay overnight at a friend's house because you don't have your special pillow? Every time you do something which negatively affects your life, or which stops you from doing something you really want to do, every time you actively compromise your life because of your insomnia, you reinforce your problem and prolong your recovery time!

Let me make one thing quite clear:

You won't get over your insomnia
until you stop making compromises for it.

Don't postpone in the hope that a time will come when you feel 'more confident'. Don't waste another day waiting for your life to start. That time will never come. At some point you have to take the plunge, you have to start saying 'yes' to invitations, you have to start making plans, you have to start doing all those things you have been avoiding because of insomnia. Life is now – start living.

From now on, keep religiously to the promises you have made as part of this programme. But in all other ways, you should act exactly as you would do if you had never had a problem with insomnia. Be warned: in the short term, this could have a negative effect on your sleep. Like a spoiled child, your insomnia may well throw a tantrum and stop you sleeping the first few times that you stand up to it. Treat it as you would a naughty child, and ignore it! Before long the message will get through: you are no longer going to tiptoe around, avoiding things which may affect your sleep, no matter how much fuss your insomnia tries to make. At some point, you *must* take a risk. This is important because when you start to take the risk of not sleeping, there will no longer be any safety to be found in avoidance behaviour and, only then, will this pattern break.

If your problem is that you cannot sleep before exciting or important events then you need to start experimenting with making fun plans yourself. Don't make these events huge elaborate affairs that might cause even the best sleeper to worry. We are just trying to get you back into the habit of making plans and of looking forward to the future without anxiety about sleep. You can start simply by organising something for the next day, something you can look forward to.

It will soon start to feel like 'the norm' to have something fun going on. Your brain will cease to categorise fun events as somehow 'special', and so they will no longer have the power to cause fear and worry. And so you relax … This is just the way life is now. Before long, a day will come when you make an elaborate plan all on your own without even *remembering* to worry about sleep.

The most important thing about this promise is to no longer contrive to avoid anxiety-producing situations. Eventually you need to *seek out* those situations, face them head on and show them who's boss! *You* are now in control of your life, *you* get to decide exactly how to spend your time, *not* your insomnia! From now on, you will do *exactly as you please* and to *hell* with your insomnia!

**From now on, your life comes first,
not your insomnia.**

And I'm going to sneak in one last rule, the 13th 'rule'.

Read This Book Often!

Read and internalise, not just the rules and the cure section, but also the consolidation chapter and the introductory sections. These will add to your understanding of your situation and will serve to motivate you when your mood is low.

THE 12 PROMISES

1.   **Spend less time in bed**

2.   **No naps**

3.   **Get up when you can't sleep**

4.   **Get up at the same time every day**

5.   **Do NOTHING in bed but sleep or sex**

6.   **Kick the pills**

7.   **Stop clock-watching**

8.   **Replace negative sleep talk with positive statements**

9.   **Let go of the search for an external miracle cure**

10. **Find a relaxation method which works for you**

11. **Find a safety net/relax into your safety thought**

12. **Put your life first**

And finally,
READ THIS BOOK OFTEN

CHAPTER ELEVEN

Synopsis

Imagine that one bright sunny day you decide to go for a walk. On turning the corner of a shady street, you find yourself dazzled by the sudden appearance of the sun from behind a tall building. You are momentarily blinded which disorients you and, for a moment, you feel a sense of dizziness and panic. Later that day, while flicking through a magazine you find there is a name for the panic which can occur on being dazzled by the sun – it is a condition known as solagoraphobia. The next day is sunny again and once again, you start to panic when you feel the sun on your face.

Searching online you find that solagoraphobia is a very common and serious condition which affects millions of people all over the world, and that there are many drugs available to treat it. Worried, you go to your doctor who gives you pills for anxiety. But the various pills she gives you either don't work or have unpleasant side-effects. The final drug she prescribes seems to work. But soon it loses its effect and you find that when you stop taking it, the anxiety returns, much worse than ever before. You are now too scared to leave the house except on a cloudy day. You then turn to alternative cures and remedies, special sunglasses and hats, none of which has any effect. Because the nervousness has worsened, you stop putting yourself in situations when it can occur. You stop going on holiday, you rarely venture out of the house between dawn and dusk. And all the while, you continue to research, finding out that your condition is misunderstood, that 'more research needs to be done', that some suffer for decades, that there is no known cure ...

How helpful was this diagnosis and treatment? Think about the effect that hearing about, and being treated for, solagoraphobia has had on the condition itself. How would you anticipate the prospect of going out on a sunny day? Are you likely to look forward to it? And, if you were ever again dazzled by the sun, how do you think you would react? Would you have any hope of curing it? What effect did hearing *this story* about solagoraphobia have on your life in general? Is it possible that you would have been better off without ever having had the 'diagnosis'?

The situation with insomnia is exactly similar to that of solagoraphobia. The only difference is that there *is* no such thing as solagoraphobia. I made the whole thing up.

Can you see that, in a similar sense, there *is* no such thing as insomnia? Insomnia is just a word we give to various different circumstances loosely involving insufficient sleep. Of course, it is true that many people do not get sufficient sleep on a regular basis and I would never belittle or ridicule the blight on your life that lack of sleep may be having. I am just trying to make you see that you do not have a 'condition', a disease that needs medical treatment.

In broad terms, I am speaking of the danger in the giving of a label. You will already be familiar with the placebo effect – the positive effect that an inactive medicine can have. You may be surprised to hear that research is now being carried out into the *nocebo effect* – the negative effect on health and behaviour of a label or diagnosis.

All that is left once the label 'insomnia' has been dropped are some nights when you didn't get enough sleep. There is no 'condition' over and above this.

To recap: this method will remedy both the poor sleep and begin to dissolve the label in the following way:

The Effortless Sleep Method:

First: achieve a solid base of good bedtime habits to ensure that a) you are really tired and sleepy when you lie down at night, and b) that bed becomes strongly associated with being asleep and *not* with lying awake, fretting. For most, *this will be all it takes* to begin sleeping normally again.

Second: transform the story you tell, to yourself and others. For chronic insomniacs the key to recovery will be the change in thoughts, the change in belief and the change in attitude – in realising that the cure is not going to come from an external source, it can only come from a change within you.

Simple isn't it? A little too simple, perhaps …

For Those Still in Doubt

If you have been suffering for some time you may feel a little dissatisfied or even disappointed in the solution I have given, especially if you were expecting a secret instant miracle cure. Is your confidence so low that summoning the motivation even to begin the programme is overwhelming? Are you suffering with sleep deprivation now, at this very moment? Or is it that memories of sleepless nights and next-day exhaustion are still fresh and raw? Such memories have a habit of clinging on and sabotaging your confidence, reminding you of how bad things can be.

But think about it: over the years there have been plenty of nights where you have actually slept quite well. It is only because those *bad* nights have caused you so much unhappiness and trouble that they have grabbed all the attention.

Now, just imagine that for all these years you had instead only focussed on the *good* nights …

Start doing it … now. From this moment, commit to focussing *only* on all that is good about your sleeping. Start telling a new story. Watch those good nights turn to good weeks, and good months. Watch your confidence grow.

Once this corner has been turned, once you have decided to take control and show your lack of fear, insomnia will never again get a stranglehold. I now sometimes challenge myself to be able to sleep in circumstances where once it would have been impossible – on the kitchen floor, in the open air, or sitting bolt upright. So, you see, I have turned the fear on its head. This is the only way that *true* recovery can occur for a chronic insomniac.

The truth is, I still obsess, just not about my sleeping problem. Now I obsess about how *well* I sleep. I obsess about how best to get my message across, about clearer, easier ways to help others to overcome their problem. It feels wonderful to say: 'I slept brilliantly last night' *and really mean it*. When there is no longer any doubt that you are recovering, when it is a *fact*, and not mere wishful thinking, your recovery will accelerate through the roof and your life will change forever. *Refuse* to be a victim any longer. You are not 'different', nor are you afflicted with a disease. You have simply developed some unhelpful habits, and *all* habits can be broken.

But it takes time …

This method is about gradually moving *away* from seeing insomnia as a disease, as a condition, as a monster. Insomnia is *not* a monster. Insomnia is not a thing at all.

This method is about gradually moving *towards* a time when seeing yourself as broken, or ill, and worrying about sleep, is a thing of the past.

Soon, the good nights will begin to far outweigh the bad nights. And eventually, the time will come when you suddenly realise you cannot remember the last time you missed a night's sleep. And finally, you will take the last step to the ultimate safety thought, a shift in attitude and belief which allows the following to be true:

I don't care whether I sleep or not.

Just think how different your life would be if missing a night of sleep hardly bothered you. Wouldn't it be wonderful if this *were* true? Try to get a sense of the way in which cultivating this belief would set you free. Can you also see that worrying so much about missing sleep only keeps you trapped? When you no longer mind whether you sleep or not, *'insomnia' can have no power over you!*

Of course, at the moment, you *do* mind. You mind very much! But notice that as you begin to improve, you cease to be so concerned about sleep. When this happens, *you are starting not to mind.* This so-called 'monster' is losing its grip, its power is diminishing. You are becoming *free,* because the ultimate freedom is in no longer caring one jot about sleep, or the lack of it.

For the Hardcore Insomniac (not for the Faint-hearted!)

Is this all *still* not what you want to hear? Still believe your condition is special, or that you have a different kind of insomnia? Still expecting to hear about some medical advance, secret herb or technique which will instantly cure you, forever? That's fine. It's your life, after all. Put this book down, try a few more remedies, waste a bit more money and come to the same realisation I did, a few more years down the line.

How much more time are you going to waste before you admit it to yourself? How much longer do you want to hang on to your insomnia? Stop having to be right, stop trying to make me wrong and embrace that which, deep down, you already suspect to be true.

> 'Advice is what we ask for when we already know the answer,
> but wish we didn't' – Erica Jong

If your response is to continue to claim 'This won't work on me' then don't be surprised when it doesn't. After all, you are still boasting about how bad and different your problem is. Believe me, your recovery will not start until this boasting stops. Do you also refuse to stick to the very easy, very basic sleep hygiene rules? If so, don't go away and say that the Effortless Sleep Method is rubbish – that it doesn't work, that you've heard it all before. *Do* it. Follow it to the letter and *then* try to rubbish it. Do it and you'll be so thrilled at your new-found ability to sleep that you will be talking about the method at parties.

You now stand at the fork in the road. One path is new and unfamiliar. It perhaps appears quite indistinct, and you may be a little unsure about where it leads. But it is the road which many others have travelled along, and those who have stayed on it have found something wonderful at the end – *they have found deep, effortless sleep.*

The other path is sure and familiar. It leads clearly off in exactly the same direction in which you have been travelling. If you continue along this path, you will continue doing exactly what you are doing, and *you will continue to get exactly what you are getting.*

The question now is: what will you do?

Will you trust me? Will you join me? Will you make the commitment?

I am waiting for you.

CHAPTER TWELVE

Q and A

Q: What if it Doesn't Work?

There is only one reason this method may not work for you – it is that you have not kept to the commitments.

This programme uses two modes of attack in the battle against insomnia. The first is to correct poor sleep habits, the other is to deal with the negative and often faulty thinking that reinforces and escalates the problem. This combined approach can work like magic and for those who really commit to the programme, their sleeping problems improve very rapidly, sometimes virtually stopping overnight. These two ways of tackling the issue correspond very roughly to short-term and chronic insomnia respectively. But the correspondence is only approximate and a person will almost always have an element of both poor sleeping habits and negative thinking. This is why the method really is a 'one fits all' solution.

If, after a few weeks, you are not seeing any benefit, then you are almost certainly not following the instructions properly.

Sometimes people report that they seem to get better initially but then run into another spell of bad sleep. When this happens it is always for the same reason – they have fallen down on the commitments of the method. They start lying in at weekends, watching television in bed, they are too often napping on the train, or they find themselves telling a stranger how bad their problem is.

If you find that you seem to relapse after some initial success, just go back to the beginning of the programme and re-commit.

Q: I accidentally Slept in or Had a Nap or Boasted about my Insomnia. Have I Ruined Everything?

Normal sleep happens through a combination of the physical conditions conducive to sleep, and a healthy dose of self-belief. The vital difference between this and many other sleep 'cures', including SR, is that these commitments *are not what 'make' the sleep happen.* They do not force sleep, they *allow* sleep. This means that a small mistake does not mean the plan is ruined, or that insomnia need return. The worst that *might* happen is that you will miss a night's sleep. If this happens, just go straight back to the programme. One lapse is really no worse than eating fish and chips while on Weight-watchers. As long as you go back to the diet the next day, there is little harm done.

Q: What if I Get Worse?

Be warned that the behavioural changes of the Effortless Sleep Method may mess with your head to start with. Letting go of your crutches, refusing to look at any more articles on insomnia, telling people what a good sleeper you are, and starting to make plans without any regard for how they will affect your sleep can sometimes play havoc with your sleep for a while. But if this happens, keep at it. The commitments of the Effortless Sleep Method have been created to make sure both of these conditions are met. The behavioural changes facilitate normal sleep, encouraging confidence in one's ability to sleep unaided, gradually producing a change in belief. Stick to the promises. Your insomnia will soon get bored with throwing a tantrum and when it does, it will have *permanently* lost much of its power over you.

Q: I have only had insomnia for a few weeks, but you tell me that for some people it goes on for 30 years. How do you know it won't take me 30 years to get over it too?

If your sleeping problem is a relatively recent occurrence, don't imagine that you will have to turn into one of those 20 or 30-year insomniacs you may come across on the online forums. *You just need to make sure that you don't make the same mistake that they do.*

There is something that keeps lifelong insomniacs in their miserable state. It is not just insomnia that unites those 20-30 year insomniacs – it is their search! The sad fact is: that quest for an external 'remedy' ensures that they will always be looking in the wrong place, and so they continue to suffer. This search constantly sends the signal to their conscious and unconscious mind that 'there is something wrong with me', and while that message is being sent, there will indeed, continue to be 'something wrong with them'.

When you direct your focus in a positive, optimistic direction, and decide to commit to doing something about your insomnia, you instantly separate from all of those chronic long-termers, and set yourself on a completely different path to them – the path to recovery.

Q: Don't tell me that I can expect a bad night from time to time. I need to believe that this will work every night, no matter what. This is the only way I will have enough faith to be able to fall asleep. How can I guarantee that I'll never have another bad night?

This thinking is an example of the catastrophising that chronic insomniacs are prone to. Just as one good night does not mean you are cured forever, so a missed night's sleep does not mean that your problem is back! This is why it is vital you accept that *one missed night is not a relapse.*

While using the Effortless Sleep Method, you may well begin sleeping better from day one, especially if you have had a previous habit of going to bed when not sleepy. But you also need to accept that from time to time, just like most of the population of the world, you may still experience a bad night. One bad night is not something that normal sleepers fear. So don't remain trapped in a pattern of panicking and catastrophising every time you miss a night's sleep.

Not minding about whether you sleep is probably the one single most important (and difficult) change in attitude that you can make. If you are in the throes of chronic insomnia, this thought may seem like an impossibility. Two years ago it would have made me angry if anyone dared suggest that I should not mind whether or not I slept. But this is one of the greatest keys to beating chronic insomnia. When you don't care whether you will sleep or not, all pressure is gone and sleep comes so much more easily. Remember

Chronic long-term insomnia is caused largely by the fear of not sleeping.

If you can *accept* that it's perfectly OK to miss the odd night then the fear loses its grip. Paradoxically, you are then more likely to be able to sleep. So reclaim your power from the beast of insomnia. Refuse to allow it to frighten you, to torment you, to ruin your life any longer.

Q: I've missed a night's sleep, it's an important day and I feel terrible. What shall I do?

The answer to this is, in short, to resolve, as best you can, to go about your life paying no attention to the fact that you have slept badly the night before.

We all have friends who seem not to suffer when they miss a night's sleep. Do you know people who think nothing of going to work after an all-night party, or who stay awake all night through choice? Why is it that some people seem not to be affected by lack of sleep, even though they must be exhausted? The answer is that they do not consider themselves to be insomniacs, and so do not add worry to the feeling of exhaustion. You may find it hard, but believe me, much of the discomfort associated with missing sleep is due to the tension and worry about how bad it feels.

After a bad night, practise allowing that tired feeling to 'be there', without focussing on it, worrying about it, judging it, or fretting about it. To do this successfully will take a bit of practice, but it will be worth the effort. First, acknowledge the *feeling*. Where is it? Really allow yourself to *feel* it, without fight or resistance, without thinking of how best to get rid of the feeling, or of what you can do to make it better. Think to yourself 'I feel really tired today, *and that's OK.*' Just accept that today it's OK to feel tired. Let that thought in. Then *let it go, and get on with your day.*

You may notice that if you have nothing particularly important to do the actual feeling of sleep deprivation seems to be much less severe. But on a day when you feel you really 'need' sleep, all you feel is intolerable misery. This happens because when you feel you really need the sleep, you are adding worry and tension to tiredness. Can you remember a time when you were completely exhausted but still happy and productive? If you can, you can feel like that again.

Sleep deprivation is *much* more bearable if you do not worry about it.

Q: How can I stay motivated to stay on the programme when I haven't slept well?

For the first few weeks, it will help if you can judge success, not by how well you have slept, but in terms of how well you have stuck to the programme. Success does not just apply to the amount of sleep you get. The truth is that whenever you make a positive change, no matter how small, you get a little better. When you get up on a Sunday at a good hour, when you resist the temptation to have a nap in the afternoon, when you are asked 'how's your insomnia?' and you answer positively, when you drop into the conversation 'I slept like a *log* last night', when you do any of these things, *you are getting better.*

The truth is, *every behavioural step in the right direction is a step towards recovery.* So if you do not sleep on any particular night then you have still made a step towards recovery *as long as you have kept to the commitments of the plan.* Think to yourself: 'I may not sleep tonight but as long as I keep up the behavioural changes, the thoughts and beliefs will follow and so, eventually, will the sleep. I am still making progress, I am still getting better.' Sleep hygiene and related behaviour are just as much a part of the problem as the lack of sleep itself. So in the early days, just be content with changing one part of the vicious circle.

Q: Nothing else has ever worked, why should I believe that this solution will be any different?

Because insomniacs have often had years of disappointment, and been told so much nonsense by so many so-called experts, they often have an automatic sceptical voice that pops in and tries to find the flaw in what they are hearing. It is a kind of 'bullsh*t detector'. The only problem is that in insomniacs it is often set way too high, giving nothing a chance. This is why, when they buy a new product, the first thing they do is to 'test' it. The thought is that because their insomnia is so severe and so predictable, they can very quickly and easily tell whether something works. So within a few days they can be sending the product back and asking for a refund. Or, more likely, that they simply put it away in some cupboard under the stairs – another reject, another failed insomnia cure.

Now I know that your mind is clever, *very* clever: it can and will search out and find any chink, any flaw in any remedy or cure. It will then exploit that weakness, focus on it and exaggerate it until the cure begins to stop working. But try to find a chink in the Effortless Sleep Method. Your mind will not find one. There is none. This programme gives you *real* confidence, not the sort of 'contrived' confidence that never lasts. You will be safe in the knowledge that basically, you can sleep – on your own, without drugs or plans or external crutches. Nothing will touch this thought, nothing will undermine this belief because you will have proved it to yourself. You may initially not like the method, but after a modicum of success you will stop looking for flaws. When you have real trust in your own ability to sleep, your mind will never again worry about trying to find chinks in the armour of this method. You will have better things to do.

- CONCLUSION-

One fateful day, months or years ago, you started having a problem sleeping. It stands to reason that if you were to recover, that recovery would begin one day too. How would you like that day to be *right now?* From this very moment, you can start to create your own future and all it will take is some common-sense behavioural changes and a shift in focus. In fact, The Effortless Sleep Method could be distilled down into two vital basic principles.

First and foremost: *keep good sleep hygiene (no excuses!)*
Second: *tell the right story*.

'What is the right story,' you ask? That's easy … the right story is the one you would like to be true. Because I promise you this

**The more you talk about how good your sleeping is,
the better it will become.**

Your recovery will begin from the *moment* you make the commitment to embark on the Effortless Sleep Method. Deciding to stop insomnia running your life is such a momentous reclaiming of power, that simply by making this decision your sleep may well improve from day one. I recovered after 15 chronic years using exactly the methods laid out in this book. If I can do it, so can you. So, whenever you feel ready to join the world of normal sleepers, make the commitment, keep to the promises, and …

… sleep well.

Appendix...

THE EFFORTLESS SLEEP RELAXATION TECHNIQUES

The Effortless Sleep
Relaxation Methods and Techniques

I have separated these nine techniques into three sections: first are three of the best relaxation methods that require additional external artificial aids. The second three are somewhat similar to standard relaxation practices with which you may already be familiar. Finally are three you won't have heard of before. These involve looking within at one's thoughts and emotions. They are the most difficult and the most effective.

When reading through this chapter, it may seem to you that there is little difference between some of these techniques. Despite this, you may find only one or all of them effective. So pick whichever you like the sound of first and try it *for a fortnight* before moving on to another. Sometimes it is the subtlest change in wording or focus which makes the difference between a method working for a particular person and not.

The most important thing to remember is that these methods should be seen as cures in themselves. *None* is likely to help if the other commitments are not in place.

The Best of The 'External' Methods

Tapping, EFT, TFT

You may find it hard to believe that tapping with your fingers on various parts of your body can have any real effect on physical or emotional problems. Take it from me – *it works!* The version of this technique that I use is EFT (Emotional Freedom Technique). EFT was derived from TFT (Thought Field Therapy), invented by American psychologist Roger Callaghan. It is a needle-free version of acupuncture based on new discoveries regarding the connection between your body's subtle energies, your emotions, and your health. Tests have shown EFT to be successful in treating countless ailments covering a huge range of emotional, health and performance issues. The theory behind it is similar to that lying behind acupuncture: energy meridians running through the body can become blocked and tapping at certain points can clear these blockages and get energy flowing properly. If this sounds too new-age for you, don't worry. The good news is that you don't need to believe the theory for this therapy to work. You don't even need to believe that it will work for it to work!

I have not reproduced the full instructions as you can find all you will need to know at www.emofree.com. This is a huge FREE source of materials where you can learn more about EFT and access hundreds of pages of resources, including a complete downloadable manual of all you will need to try out this technique. It can be used throughout the day as preparation for bedtime, or when you awaken and cannot get back to sleep.

Meditation

Meditation is known to create feelings of peace and harmony in the body and mind and is used to encourage emotional and spiritual growth. It has also been shown to aid concentration, productivity, creativity and even benefit your personal relationships. But besides all this, meditation can also have an incredible effect on your sleep. In particular, regular meditation can cut the time taken to fall asleep drastically.

If you do fancy learning to meditate then it may be best to attend a class in order to get some initial instruction but you can also practise on your own by using one of the following simple techniques:

1)   Focus on the feeling of your breath
2)   Repeat a meaningless mantra such as *shirr-ring*

If you wish to meditate to make your 'background state' more relaxed, you should sit in the traditional cross-legged posture, in a chair, or in any upright position that is comfortable. It is important to keep your back straight to prevent your mind from becoming sluggish or sleepy.

However, if you wish to use meditation to *send* you to sleep at night, either breathing meditation or mantra meditation can be done lying down in bed until you fall asleep.

Focusing on the Breath

Sit or lie comfortably for a few minutes. Close your eyes and turn your attention to your breathing. Breathe naturally, preferably through the nostrils, without attempting to control or interfere with the breath. Try to become aware of the sensation of the breath as it enters and leaves the nostrils. This sensation is the object of meditation. Try *gently* to concentrate on it to the exclusion of everything else.

It will be tempting to follow the different thoughts as they arise, but resist this temptation and remain focused on the sensation of the breath. If you discover that your mind has wandered and is following your thoughts, gently return your focus to the breath.

Using a Mantra

If using a mantra, it is important to make sure that the word used is meaningless, otherwise it may create concepts, associations and pictures in the mind. Sit or lie comfortably for a few minutes. Close your eyes for about half a minute, then open them again. Notice that when your eyes were closed, some thoughts arose into your consciousness. Think about how gently and subtly these thoughts arose. In just the same subtle and effortless way, allow the mantra to appear in your mind and start gently repeating it to yourself. Do not force the sound of the mantra or make it a particular pitch or frequency.

Again, resist the temptation to follow the different thoughts that may arise. If you discover that your mind has wandered, and that the mantra has stopped, gently return your focus to the mantra and begin repeating it again. If the mantra starts to change, sound different, speed up, slow down, or turn somersaults, *let it*. Make no attempt to keep the mantra 'pure'. This would mean using too much effort and concentration.

In both mantra meditation and breathing meditation, the point is to *rest* your mind on the target (the breath or the mantra) without strong concentration. Don't make a big effort to keep the target in mind; this is not about *using* your mind, it is about *watching* your mind. If thoughts come up, let them be. Do not engage with them, do not judge them or yourself, just watch them. In meditation, no thought is wrong.

Both of these methods are ideal for calming an overactive mind. If busy thoughts are keeping you awake at night, try to perfect one of these methods. Both have a very similar effect.

Meditation using Binaural Beats

However, if you do not have the discipline to learn to meditate, or you simply find it difficult to still your mind, there is a truly *effortless* route to the perfect meditative state. The quickest and easiest way to meditate is to use binaural beats meditation recordings. Binaural beats are produced when a person listens to different sound frequencies in the left and right ear, so producing 'beats'. The resultant frequency has the capacity to take the listener into a profoundly deep state of meditation within minutes simply by relaxing in a quiet environment, closing your eyes and wearing headphones.

Binaural beats meditations have the benefit of being able to be used even when it is not possible to find a quiet moment in the day. All you need is a pair of headphones or ear-buds. The odd door slamming, barking dog or murmur from the television set is not going to disturb this type of meditation. There are many companies now offering meditation recordings using binaural beats. Among these are Holosync, Hemisync and Perfect Meditation. I personally find Holosync (www.centerpointe.com) the most effective, simply because the quality of the recording seems superior to some of the cheaper types. You may find that Holosync works best if used to calm your general background state, rather than as a bedtime sleep-inducer. However, I have found that each time I start a new, stronger level of Holosync, I find it impossible to stay awake, even when sitting up. Sadly, this rather pleasant side-effect wears off after a few listens.

Brain Entrainment to Relax

Using the same technology as the binaural beats described above, brainwave entrainment recordings can be used to evoke all manner of relaxed states of mind and body.

Neurologists have discovered that if sound stimuli are precisely timed to the electrical activity of the brain, brainwave patterns can actually be altered and the mental state of a person can be changed. As an example, someone who is wide awake may start to feel relaxed and drowsy when given a stimulus corresponding to a relaxed brainwave pattern. This technology is now over 70 years old and brainwave entrainment is now widely used for a variety of purposes to train the brain to a particular mental state. It has become so widely used that many clinical EEG units come with entrainment devices.

I have created a range of brain entrainment Sleep Tool recordings designed specifically for insomnia. Check the website for details.

A Note About the Effortless Sleep Booster Tool

The Effortless Sleep Booster Tool is an SMR brainwave entrainment recording. Long-term insomniacs often seem to find SMR (sensory motor rhythm) recordings more helpful than specific relaxation or sleep induction sessions. SMR recordings rend to make it easier for you to *learn* to sleep in the future, rather than being directly relaxing in themselves. For this reason, I recommend listening to the Booster Tool alongside learning the method itself. However, if you are like me, you will find SMR recordings like the Sleep Booster Tool as relaxing as many sleeping medications with none of the side-effects.

The Sleep Booster Tool forms part of the Effortless Sleep Tools pack which is included in my complete online programme. These tools are also available as a separate package, for those who have already purchased this book.

You can order these sleep tools at a special price from www.sashastephens.com/discount.

Best of the 'Standard' Relaxation Techniques

The following three techniques are not ones which I personally have found helpful, but have been reported by others as extremely effective. If you are one of those who needs to give your mind something to 'do' then try one of the following techniques:

Retracing Your Steps

When you lie down and turn out the light, relax and turn your attention inwards. Think about the events of the day. Visualise what you were doing just before you got into bed. What did you do immediately before this? Retrace the events of the day, playing them back to yourself in your mind. Don't rush. Visualise in detail, remembering what was said and heard, and what you saw at the time. Carry on, going backwards through all the events of the day until you end up at the point at which you woke up.

This not only focuses your mind on something other than sleep, allowing you to drift off, it can also be a very good way to 'put the day to bed', to let go of the day's events and lessen thoughts which may otherwise plague your sleep. Sometimes a thought may pop up which requires action, or stimulates further thoughts – you may realise you have forgotten to do something today, or that something important needs to be done, or thought about tomorrow. If such thoughts keep you awake, have a pen and paper next to the bed on which to scribble anything which needs your future attention, and tell yourself you will deal with it tomorrow.

Retrace your thoughts

Similar to this is to retrace your thoughts. Start by focussing on your current thought and follow your train of thought backwards trying to remember which thought led to the present one. Then remember what you were thinking to inspire that thought, and so on, back and back, retracing your thoughts further into the past.

And keep doing it!

This technique is slightly more difficult than retracing the day's events, but for this very reason it is particularly effective for distracting your mind from worrying about sleeping, allowing you to drift off into sleep.

For goodness sake, do not try it once for five minutes, find yourself still awake and conclude that it doesn't work. This needs to be done until you fall asleep. And like most other techniques, its effectiveness increases the more often you do it.

The body scan

Do a 'body scan'. Starting at the top of your head, gently allow your mind to focus on each part of your body. Feel the tension which is there, and allow it to release. Go through the body, not moving from head, to shoulders, to arms and hands, but *slowly* by relaxing your forehead, your eyebrows, your eyesockets, your scalp, chin, upper lip, lower lip, jawbones etc. Not only is this deeply relaxing, it is also very boring! The combination of boredom and relaxation will often mean that you will be asleep before you have got half way down your body.

The New 'Effortless Sleep Techniques'

I particularly recommend that you experiment with all of this last set. They can be tricky to get right but these more unusual techniques have the most profound effect. All are designed to send you to sleep at night, even on the most difficult and high-pressured nights.

Keeping Your Focus on the Body

If you pay attention to the way you feel when you are very drowsy, or have just woken up, you will notice that your attention is located in your body, not on anything external. Rather than trying to watch your thoughts, or focussing hard on relaxing on a particular part of your body, try focussing *gently* in a very general way on your body. Try to feel its 'energy', its warmth, the actual way that it, as a whole, seems to feel to you.

You will begin to feel warm, glowing, and will relax naturally and without effort. It's a lovely feeling. Let your thoughts do whatever they want. Do not try to stop them, follow them or engage with them in any way. You will start to drift off very soon. From time to time a troublesome thought may pop in to take your attention and rouse you a little, or you may suddenly become aware with a little jolt. If this happens, don't let it panic you; just *gently* return your attention to the feeling of the warm energy field of your body, and let the thoughts carry on again. Although this appears to be yet another type of meditation, it is not designed to calm your overactive mind. Rather, most people find it deeply *physically* relaxing.

'Doing Nothing'

This is my personal favourite of all the relaxation techniques here, if it can be called a technique. It is more difficult than it sounds but I thoroughly recommend that you make an effort to get the hang of it. Once mastered it is the most valuable relaxation tool there is. After all, this is exactly what the majority of really good sleepers do every night. It is the technique I still use to this day. It seems to be the most effective when you are feeling quite sleepy and drowsy already, and seems to prevent the 'waking' effects of 'trying' to fall asleep. At first sight it seems like another form of meditation. But the effect is very different.

Lie down, turn out the light and do *nothing.*
It is important not to 'try' to do nothing.
Do not avoid thinking about sleep, nor try to think about sleep.
Do not concentrate on 'doing nothing', or on anything at all.
If thoughts arise, let them. Don't engage with them, or try to stop them.
In other words, just 'do' nothing at all.

Your body may respond in all sorts of ways including relaxing and getting drowsy, or even by tensing up, jerking or thinking, but this is fine so long as you do not 'try' to relax or get drowsy, that you do not 'try' to stop tensing up or stop thinking. If you start feeling drowsy and sleepy, don't try to hang on to that feeling, don't try to keep your body in that drowsy place. Leave your thoughts, feelings, emotions, and body to their own devices. Let your body and mind do whatever it wants to and do not intervene, positively or negatively. Just allow everything. This is difficult and counter-intuitive at first because we are so used to 'doing' something in every moment of our waking lives. But persevere, and you will become better at it.

You will eventually become aware of how much you are still actively intervening with the thoughts and functioning of your body, and you will go deeper, allowing more and intervening even less. There is always less you can be doing, and when this 'doing' becomes as minimised as possible, profoundly small, I guarantee you *will* fall asleep. I describe this as *profoundly* doing nothing!

If you are one of those unfortunate people who find themselves beginning to wake up as soon as they become aware of becoming drowsy, then this will be the ideal technique for you. If it seems that it's not working one night, know that *sleep often comes suddenly when using this technique*, without any conscious increase in relaxation. You may suddenly find yourself awake having been asleep for some time, without ever having noticed yourself becoming drowsier.

The Ultimate Technique

For those of you who are still protesting that nothing works, I have something especially for you. This tool is the most powerful weapon against insomnia on those nights when all the guidelines have been followed, all seems well but you simply aren't able to sleep. Again it takes a little while to get the hang of, but persevere – it will transform your insomnia and is actually a very useful tool which can be used to help depression, anxiousness, anger, guilt, and even physical symptoms such as back pain. I have even relieved a nasty hangover with this technique!

I came up with it after years of meditation involving 'watching the breath' and also from learning the Sedona Method. (You can learn more about it at www.sedona.com.) The Sedona Method is one of the most effective self-help methods available and I have found it incredibly beneficial for dealing with all manner of emotional issues. But I found that like many other of the more effective self-help methods available, it helped my life in a myriad of ways, but it never got rid of the insomnia. It seemed that this problem was so set, so solid, so much part of my life that no technique could touch it. It was then that I had one of the brainwaves which changed everything.

For most people, the simple sleep hygiene rules and relaxation techniques offered in section one are enough to make a huge difference to their sleep and for many this advice alone will cure the problem for good. But for the long term insomniac, the problem has gone beyond bad sleep habits. It has become about worry, lack of belief, and *fear*.

It is fear which makes the problem of insomnia so persistent. For many people, all it takes to cause panic is the thought that they aren't going to be able to sleep, sending adrenaline levels sky high and keeping them awake. For these people, the fear is so entrenched and the pattern is so set in stone that even the word 'sleep' can set off something approaching a phobic reaction. So for many, particularly long-term sufferers, it is literally the fear of not sleeping that stops them from sleeping and because they know this, they end up not just with fear, but fear of fear, and fear of fear of fear. A vicious circle then sets in whereby the fear stops the sleeping and the lack of sleeping reinforces the fear. This sort of mechanism contributes greatly to the creation and reinforcement of long-term chronic insomnia.

But hope is at hand! I'm now going to tell you about the most powerful and effective technique in my arsenal – one that will actually use fear itself to help you sleep. OK. How do you deal with something you are afraid of?

You fight it? You run away?

Fight or flight is the classic response. But what if the thing you are afraid of is anxiety itself? If you choose to fight it head on, you just make it persist even longer. The battle itself draws attention to the fact that you are fighting an enemy; reinforcing the idea keeps the anxiety in place. But if you choose to run away you are showing just how much you fear it, and it comes back to torment you, again and again.

There is a third option: we are going to work on *neutralising* the fear. How do you neutralise anything? – you bring in its opposite. The opposite of running from fear, or fighting fear, is *welcoming* – if you could really welcome fear, you would literally no longer be afraid of it and it would evaporate. This is exactly how we are going to tackle our fear of not sleeping.

If you are familiar with relaxing or meditating by watching the breath then you will know that this involves focussing the mind on the physical sensation of breathing. If not, this may be a good place to start to get you used to focussing on bodily sensations. It may be easiest to get used to the practice of watching the breath before moving on to this technique.

But there is one problem with this method of meditation; because the mind focuses *on* the breath, it still involves a separation of body and mind and the breath remains somehow distinct from 'you'. I now want you to try something different. Try shifting your focus from *watching* the breath to *being* the breath. Allow your sense of 'I', your awareness almost to merge with the breath. This may sound a little strange but it is really very easy. If you find this difficult you can help by saying silently to yourself *I am the breath, I am the breath.* You should find this instantly very relaxing and you may even feel as if your body and mind are melting into each other, or have become indistinguishable.

Now you need to try this with your fear of insomnia. Bring up an anxiety-inducing thought now. As the fear arises do not fight it, allow it to be there, really *feel* it. Then move one step further, *allow* it to be there. *Welcome* it. This is very similar to the Sedona Method so far. But now, finally, I want you to do just as you did when you focused on *being* the breath. You need to *be* the fear. Slide your awareness *into* the fear, become one with it. If you like, say to yourself *I am fear, I am fear.*

See how the fear transmutes! See how it dissolves! See how it is neutralised! And isn't this the most relaxing thing you have ever done? The fear transforms and becomes revealed for what it really is – a phantom, a nothing. Just as the fear of a darkened room is neutralised by the clarity offered by turning on the light, so clarity is offered by looking head on at the fear of not sleeping. Allow it to neutralise without running, fighting, avoiding or changing the subject, but looking head on at that fear and welcoming it in.

Feel your fear, allow it, welcome it, BE it.
Feel your thoughts, allow them, welcome them, BE them.
Feel your feelings, allow them, welcome them, BE them.

Anything you can truly welcome can hold no fear for you.
You cannot fear something if you can truly welcome it.

Thus your fear of not sleeping will end up being your best friend. Every fear, every tension gives you another opportunity to relax in a more profound way than ever before. If you can master this tool it will change your sleep, and your life!

But I'm afraid to even try it. What if even 'the ultimate' technique doesn't work on me? Then where will I be?

Then this is the perfect technique for you! Because you have a very clear cut feeling to work on, you have the perfect place to start. Sit with that feeling of fear of trying, and welcome and *be* it, welcome the feeling that you are different and *be* it, welcome the worry that this won't work on you and *be* that feeling! Whatever it is, *be* it and it will transform. This tool is truly amazing because even when you don't believe it will work, even when you think your problem is different from the whole world, whatever the thought, fear or belief you have is the gateway to a deeper relaxation and peaceful thoughts and *sleep*!

© *Sasha Stephens 2010*

Where to go from here?

Do you have questions? Are you wondering how to move on to the next stage of your recovery? Would you like to become not a good sleeper, but a *great* sleeper?

You will find more advanced sleep wisdom and all your questions answered in Sasha Stephens' follow-up book

The Effortless Sleep Companion

Available now from Amazon, Barnes and Noble
and from all good bookshops.

Also coming in December 2013 by Sasha Stephens

Bedtime Stories for Insomniacs

My sleep products are available at greatly reduced prices to readers. Visit www.sashastephens.com/discount to access the special prices. This page is hidden from normal view and the address is made available only to readers of this book.

Personal sleep therapy consultations with Sasha by email, Skype and in person are sometimes available.

Just visit www.sashastephens.com or www.effortless-sleep.com to find out more.